Map Key

P9-BZB-374

Trail Name	Page

Part 1 SOUTH
California Border to Mount Thielsen

1 California Border to Observation
Peak [*Day hike, Out-and-back,
6 miles*] 20

2 Grouse Gap to Siskiyou Peak
[*Day hike, Out-and-back, 5.2 miles*] 25

3 OR 99 to Pilot Rock [*Day hike,
Out-and-back, 9.2 miles*] 30

4 Sky Lakes Wilderness [*Day hike/
1–2 nights, Out-and-back, 23.8 miles*] 36

5 OR 62 to Pumice Flat [*Day hike,
Out-and-back, 15 miles*] 42

6 OR 62 to Crater Lake Rim
[*Day hike/1 night, Point-to-point,
4.3 miles*] 47

7 Crater Lake Rim [*Day hike,
Point-to-point, 6.4 miles*] 52

8 Mount Thielsen Loop
[*1–2 nights, Loop, 21.6 miles*] 58

9 Tipsoo Peak and Maidu Lake
[*2 nights, Out-and-back, 30.4 miles*] 64

Part 2 CENTRAL
Willamette Pass to Santiam Pass

10 Rosary Lakes to Maiden Peak
Shelter [*Day hike/1 night, Out-and-
back, 11.6 miles*] 72

11 Mink Lake Basin [*1–2 nights,
Out-and-back, 24 miles*] 76

12 Wickiup Plain to Sisters Mirror
Lake [*Day hike/1 night, Loop,
15.1 miles*] 81

13 Obsidian Loop [*Day hike/1–2 nights,
Out-and-back, 15.9 miles*] 86

14 Lava Camp Lake to Collier Glacier
View [*Day hike/1 night, Out-and-back,
14.8 miles*] 92

Trail Name	Page

Part 2 CENTRAL (*continued*)
Willamette Pass to Santiam Pass

15 Little Belknap Crater [*Day hike,
Out-and-back, 4.8 miles*] 98

16 Three-Fingered Jack [*Day hike/
1 night, Loop, 9.5 miles*] 102

Part 3 NORTH
Mount Jefferson to Columbia River

17 Pamelia Lake to Shale Lake Loop
[*1–2 nights, Loop, 19 miles*] 110

18 Jefferson Park [*Day hike/1 night,
Out-and-back, 14.9 miles*] 116

19 Breitenbush Lake to Park Butte
[*Day hike/1 night, Out-and-back, 7 miles*]
122

20 Olallie Lake to Upper Lake
[*Day hike, Out-and-back, 4.6 miles*] 129

21 Little Crater Lake to
Timothy Lake [*Day hike/1 night,
Out-and-back, 4.4 miles*] 135

22 Twin Lakes Loop [*Day hike/1 night,
Loop, 4–8.5 miles*] 140

23 Barlow Pass to Timberline Lodge
[*Day hike/1 night, Out-and-back,
10 miles*] 145

24 Timberline Lodge to Paradise
Park [*Day hike/1 night, Out-and-back,
13 miles*] 150

25 Ramona Falls to Sandy River Loop
[*Day hike/1 night, Loop, 13.7 miles*] 158

26 Lost Lake to Buck Peak [*Day hike/
1 night, Loop, 16 miles*] 166

27 Chinidere Mountain
[*Day hike, Loop, 4 miles*] 172

28 Eagle Creek to Benson Plateau
Loop [*1–2 nights, Loop, 29.2 miles*] 178

Other Titles of Interest

60 Hikes within 60 Miles: Portland by Paul Gerald

The Best in Tent Camping: Oregon by Jeanne Pyle and Paul Gerald

The Best in Tent Camping: Washington by Jeanne Pyle

One Night Wilderness Portland by Douglas Lorain

Backpacking Oregon by Douglas Lorain

Outdoor Navigation with GPS by Stephen W. Hinch

Hikers' and Backpackers' Guide for Treating Medical Emergencies
by Patrick Brighton, MD

For other outdoor titles from Wilderness Press and Menasha Ridge
Press, visit **www.wildernesspress.com** and **www.menasharidge.com.**

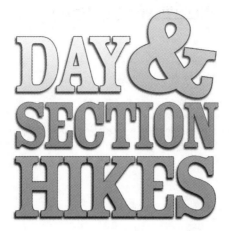

DAY & SECTION HIKES

Pacific Crest Trail
OREGON

PAUL GERALD

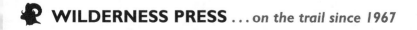

WILDERNESS PRESS ... *on the trail since 1967*

Day & Section Hikes Pacific Crest Trail: Oregon

2nd EDITION 2012
   3rd printing 2015

Front cover photos copyright © 2012 by Paul Gerald
Interior photos by the author
Maps and elevation profiles: Scott McGrew, Paul Gerald, and Steve Jones
Cover design and interior design: Ian Szymkowiak (Palace Press International)
Editor: Laura Shauger

ISBN 978-0-89997-689-1

Manufactured in the United States of America

Published by: **Wilderness Press**
               Keen Communications
               2204 First Avenue South, Suite 102
               Birmingham, AL 35233
               (800) 443-7227
               info@wildernesspress.com
               www.wildernesspress.com

Visit our website for a complete listing of our books and for ordering information.
Distributed by Publishers Group West

Cover photos: Main: Observation Peak (Hike 1); *top:* Wickiup Plain (Hike 12)

SAFETY NOTICE: Although Wilderness Press and the author have made every attempt to ensure that the information in this book is accurate at press time, they are not responsible for any loss, damage, injury, or inconvenience that may occur to anyone while using this book. You are responsible for your own safety and health while in the wilderness. The fact that a trail is described in this book does not mean that it will be safe for you. Be aware that trail conditions can change from day to day. Always check local conditions, know your own limitations, and consult a map.

Dedication

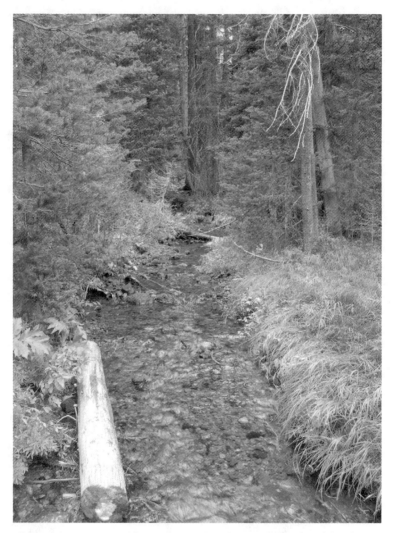

The PCT crosses Dutton Creek on the way to the Crater Lake Rim (Hike 6).

Table of Contents

Overview Map   inside front cover

Map Key   i

Acknowledgments   ix

Preface   xi

Top 5 Hikes by Category   xiii

Introduction   1

  How to Use This Guidebook   1

  Weather   5

  Water   6

  Clothing   7

  The Ten Essentials   8

  First-Aid   8

  Hiking with Children   9

  General Safety   9

  Animal and Plant Hazards   11

  Tips for Enjoying the PCT in Oregon   14

  Backcountry Advice   15

  Trail Etiquette   17

PART 1: SOUTH   19
CALIFORNIA BORDER TO MOUNT THIELSEN

1   California Border to Observation Peak
    [Day hike, Out-and-back, 6 miles]   20

2   Grouse Gap to Siskiyou Peak   [Day hike, Out-and-back, 5.2 miles]   25

3   OR 99 to Pilot Rock   [Day hike, Out-and-back, 9.2 miles]   30

4   Sky Lakes Wilderness
    [Day hike/1–2 nights, Out-and-back, 23.8 miles]   36

5   OR 62 to Pumice Flat   [Day hike, Out-and-back, 15 miles]   42

6   OR 62 to Crater Lake Rim
    [*Day hike/1 night, Point-to-point, 4.3 miles*]   47

7   Crater Lake Rim [*Day hike, Point-to-point, 6.4 miles*]   52

8   Mount Thielsen Loop [*1–2 nights, Loop, 21.6 miles*]   58

9   Tipsoo Peak and Maidu Lake [*2 nights, Out-and-back, 30.4 miles*] 64

PART 2: CENTRAL   71
WILLAMETTE PASS TO SANTIAM PASS

10 Rosary Lakes to Maiden Peak Shelter
    [*Day hike/1 night, Out-and-back, 11.6 miles*]   72

11 Mink Lake Basin [*1–2 nights, Out-and-back, 24 miles*]   76

12 Wickiup Plain to Sisters Mirror Lake
    [*Day hike/1 night, Loop, 15.1 miles*]   81

13 Obsidian Loop [*Day hike/1–2 nights, Out-and-back, 15.9 miles*]   86

14 Lava Camp Lake to Collier Glacier View
    [*Day hike/1 night, Out-and-back, 14.8 miles*]   92

15 Little Belknap Crater [*Day hike, Out-and-back, 4.8 miles*]   98

16 Three-Fingered Jack [*Day hike/1 night, Loop, 9.5 miles*]   102

PART 3: NORTH   109
MOUNT JEFFERSON TO COLUMBIA RIVER

17 Pamelia Lake to Shale Lake Loop [*1–2 nights, Loop, 19 miles*]   110

18 Jefferson Park [*Day hike/1 night, Out-and-back, 14.9 miles*]   116

19 Breitenbush Lake to Park Butte
    [*Day hike/1 night, Out-and-back, 7 miles*]   122

20 Olallie Lake to Upper Lake [*Day hike, Out-and-back, 4.6 miles*]   129

21 Little Crater Lake to Timothy Lake
    [*Day hike/1 night, Out-and-back, 4.4 miles*]   135

22 Twin Lakes Loop [*Day hike/1 night, Loop, 4–8.5 miles*]   140

23 Barlow Pass to Timberline Lodge
    [*Day hike/1 night, Out-and-back, 10 miles*]   145

24 Timberline Lodge to Paradise Park
    [*Day hike/1 night, Out-and-back, 13 miles*]   150

25 Ramona Falls to Sandy River Loop
    [*Day hike/1 night, Loop, 13.7 miles*]   158

26 Lost Lake to Buck Peak [*Day hike/1 night, Loop, 16 miles*]   166

27 Chinidere Mountain [*Day hike, Loop, 4 miles*]   172

28 Eagle Creek to Benson Plateau Loop
    [*1–2 nights, Loop, 29.2 miles*]   178

Appendix A: Hikes by Category   187

Appendix B: Contacts   188

Appendix C: Hike Agencies   190

Index   193

About the Author   199

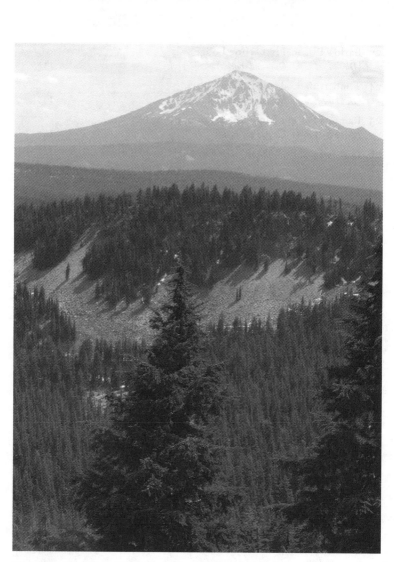

View of Mount McLoughlin in Sky Lakes Wilderness (Hike 4)

Acknowledgments

THIS WHOLE PCT THING, for me, started with my friend Corky Corcoran. He's the one who told me he was hiking across Oregon and asked if I wanted to go. That led to my quitting my job at an insurance company, selling off a bunch of my stuff, giving up my apartment, and spending four weeks in the woods. That trip ultimately led to the first edition of this book, which came out in 2007. For that one, I also thank the Fainos, Steve Moellering and his wife Diana, the Towanda Clan, Craig Schuhmann, the Thursday Night Boys, Jean Nelson, Beth McNeil, Jane Garbisch, Jim Sifferle, and Steve Queen.

Also, some fellow guidebook authors and their work must be acknowledged, because they helped fill in some gaps when I was sitting at my desk in November, wishing I had taken better notes back in August. Jeffrey P. Schaeffer and Andy Selters wrote *Pacific Crest Trail,* the definitive work for thru-hiking the PCT, and I leaned heavily on their Oregon–Washington volume. William Sullivan's *100 Hikes* series was helpful, as was Megan McMorris's *Oregon Hiking.* And if you see anything here about why a thing or place is called what it's called, that came straight from the incomparable *Oregon Geographical Names,* sixth edition, by Lewis A. McArthur.

For this second edition, a whole new batch of helpers emerged, mainly to review the text and make sure I wasn't directing anybody off of a cliff. They included David Grimes at Crater Lake National Park, as well as Forest Service staffers Christy Martin, Mark Ellis, and Randy Menke. The bulk of the help came from the lovely people at the Pacific Crest Trail Association, starting with Executive Director Liz Bergeron and regional coordinators Ian Nelson and Dana Hendricks. Eventually these section volunteers looked at my scribbles: Kate Beardsley, Bill Carpenter, Brian Briggs, Paul Martin Smith,

Ernie Strahm, Roberta Cobb, Ron Goodwin, Kim Owen, Leif Hoven, and John Vhay. And it was really cool to run into Isaac Daniel on the trail in Three Sisters.

If I missed anybody, it's only because my brain doesn't work right—too much time sleeping on the ground, I suppose.

Preface

IT'S USUALLY ABOUT THE THIRD DAY OF A TRIP when I start to feel comfortable. The first day I'm tired, the second I feel dirty, but somewhere around the third I start to adjust. My muscles get the hang of it, I get into the rhythm of the hiking life, and a plunge in a lake fulfills the purpose of a shower. That's when the trail mind kicks in, and from there on out, life gets simpler and simpler, the senses more and more open, the days grander and grander.

It's my sincere hope that this book will lead you down the same path. If you've never hiked much or never backpacked, what you're holding can be a key to getting started. You could begin with some easy hikes, build up to an overnighter, maybe string a few together for a longer trip, and soon find yourself comfortable exploring Oregon's wondrous Pacific Crest Trail—or not. You can also use this book to day hike to the trail's highlights. And if you're an experienced hiker or backpacker, I hope this book will give you some ideas for places to go that you didn't know about.

Either way, another goal of mine is to bring you a step or two into the world of the PCT. It isn't just a trail; it's a subculture, a tribe, a way of life, a state of mind. It's a whole new way of looking at places. For example, we all know about Timberline Lodge, and we all know about Crater Lake. And we think of it as, say, a five-hour drive between the two. What I want you to do is see these places as a long-distance PCT hiker sees them: as about a two-week walk during which you will skirt the edge of towering peaks like Mount Thielsen, pass through glorious meadows near the Three Sisters, plunge into the lakes of the Olallie Basin, and slog over peak after ridge after butte. That's why, throughout this book, I've tried to tell you what a thru-hiker thinks of a place, or how many "trail miles" it is between points. Who knows? You might get so hooked you decide to hike all the way across Oregon; nothing would make me happier.

Writing a book is frankly not a lot of fun. Researching it? Sure. Driving around the state, writing off your expenses, going on hikes, camping out, dragging friends out with you, making new ones, seeing favorite places again, finding new ones . . . all wonderful. Sitting for hours at your desk, with the November rain lashing the windows and nobody around but you and the computer and a pile of notes, maps, and photos? Not so fun. Hurts the neck too.

But as I write these chapters and sort through these photos, my mind wanders back onto the trail; it also has a fine habit of forgetting the fatigue, filth, and pain. I remember the butterflies swarming around the Twin Lakes, the waterfalls around Paradise Park, the clouds swirling around Mount Jefferson, the sunset from Observation Peak, the coyote at Timothy Lake, the elk at Crater Lake, and all the fine people I met along the way. Sometimes it all becomes a warm, comfortable blur that takes in the whole state—a single trail, a single experience that stretches from the Siskiyous to the Columbia River, all the way across this amazing state we're so lucky to call home.

That's the magic of the PCT, and this book is an invitation to join me on that adventure.

Top 5 Hikes by Category

Most Scenic Hikes

7   Crater Lake Rim (*page* 52)

12 Wickiup Plain to Sisters Mirror Lake (*page* 81)

13 Obsidian Loop (*page* 86)

19 Breitenbush Lake to Park Butte (*page* 122)

24 Timberline Lodge to Paradise Park (*page* 150)

Most Difficult Hikes

8   Mount Thielsen Loop (*page* 58)

9   Tipsoo Peak and Maidu Lake (*page* 64)

16 Three-Fingered Jack (*page* 102)

24 Timberline Lodge to Paradise Park (*page* 150)

28 Eagle Creek to Benson Plateau Loop (*page* 178)

Easiest Hikes

1   California Border to Observation Peak (*page* 20)

7   Crater Lake Rim (*page* 52)

11 Mink Lake Basin (*page* 76)

20 Olallie Lake to Upper Lake (*page* 129)

21 Little Crater Lake to Timothy Lake (*page* 135)

Best-Maintained Trails

10 Rosary Lakes to Maiden Peak Shelter (*page* 72)

18 Jefferson Park (*page* 116)

21 Little Crater Lake to Timothy Lake (*page* 135)

22 Twin Lakes Loop (*page* 140)

24 Timberline Lodge to Paradise Park (*page* 150)

Best for Solitude

1   California Border to Observation Peak (*page* 20)

5   OR 62 to Pumice Flat (*page* 42)

9   Tipsoo Peak and Maidu Lake (*page* 64)

11 Mink Lake Basin (*page* 76)

26 Lost Lake to Buck Peak (*page* 166)

Best for Children

10 Rosary Lakes to Maiden Peak Shelter (*page* 72)

20 Olallie Lake to Upper Lake (*page* 129)

21 Little Crater Lake to Timothy Lake (*page* 135)

22 Twin Lakes Loop (*page* 140)

27 Chinidere Mountain (*page* 172)

WILDFLOWER HIKES

12 Wickiup Plain to Sisters Mirror Lake (*page* 81)

13 Obsidian Loop (*page* 86)

18 Jefferson Park (*page* 116)

23 Barlow Pass to Timberline Lodge (*page* 145)

24 Timberline Lodge to Paradise Park (*page* 150)

WILDLIFE HIKES

1 California Border to Observation Peak (*page* 20)

4 Sky Lakes Wilderness (*page* 36)

5 OR 62 to Pumice Flat (*page* 42)

12 Wickiup Plain to Sisters Mirror Lake (*page* 81)

26 Lost Lake to Buck Peak (*page* 166)

BEST FOR A SNOWSHOE OR SKI TRIP IN WINTER

5 OR 62 to Pumice Flat (*page* 42)

7 Crater Lake Rim (*page* 52)

10 Rosary Lakes to Maiden Peak Shelter (*page* 72)

22 Twin Lakes Loop (*page* 140)

23 Barlow Pass to Timberline Lodge (*page* 145)

HIKES WITH DOGS

1 California Border to Observation Peak (*page* 20)

10 Rosary Lakes to Maiden Peak Shelter (*page* 72)

20 Olallie Lake to Upper Lake (*page* 129)

21 Little Crater Lake to Timothy Lake (*page* 135)

22 Twin Lakes Loop (*page* 140)

STEEP HIKES

6 OR 62 to Crater Lake Rim (*page* 47)

8 Mount Thielsen Loop (*page* 58)

9 Tipsoo Peak and Maidu Lake (*page* 64)

19 Breitenbush Lake to Park Butte (*page* 122)

27 Chinidere Mountain (*page* 172)

FAIRLY FLAT HIKES

5 OR 62 to Pumice Flat (*page* 42)

11 Mink Lake Basin (*page* 76)

12 Wickiup Plain to Sisters Mirror Lake (*page* 81)

20 Olallie Lake to Upper Lake (*page* 129)

21 Little Crater Lake to Timothy Lake (*page* 135)

Introduction

How to Use This Guidebook

I'M NOT JUST A GUIDEBOOK AUTHOR; I also read and use them. So I know the temptation to skip over all this introductory material, telling yourself, "Yeah, yeah, I got it. Let's get to the hikes." But this stuff is really helpful. We want you to get the most out of this book and its maps, profiles, and GPS data. So take a few moments to read through this section; you'll appreciate it later.

THE OVERVIEW MAP AND KEY

Use the overview map on the inside front cover to assess the exact location of each hike's primary trailhead. Each hike number appears on the overview map, on the key facing that map, and in the table of contents. Flipping through the book, you can easily locate a hike's full profile by watching for the hike number at the top of the first page of its description.

The book is organized by region as indicated in the table of contents. The hikes within each region are noted as one-way day hikes, loop day hikes, or overnight loop hikes (see page vii). A map legend that details the symbols found on trail maps appears on the inside back cover.

TRAIL MAPS

Each hike contains a detailed map that shows the trailhead, the route, significant features, facilities, and topographic landmarks such as creeks, overlooks, and peaks. The author gathered map data by carrying a Garmin GPSMap 60CS while hiking. This data was downloaded into National Geographic's TOPO! program and processed by expert cartographers to produce the highly accurate maps found in this book. Each trailhead's GPS coordinates are included at the end of each profile.

Elevation Profiles

Corresponding directly to the trail map, each hike contains a detailed elevation profile. The elevation profile provides a quick look at the trail's steepness, enabling you to visualize how it rises and falls. To understand the profiles, note the number of feet between each tick mark on the vertical axis (the height scale).

GPS Trailhead Coordinates

To collect accurate map data, each trail was hiked with a handheld Garmin GPS unit. Data collected was then downloaded and plotted onto a digital USGS topo map. In addition to rendering a highly specific trail outline, this book includes the GPS coordinates for each trailhead in two formats: latitude/longitude and Universal Transverse Mercator (UTM). Latitude/longitude coordinates tell you where you are by locating a point west (latitude) of the zero-degree meridian line that passes through Greenwich, England, and north or south of the zero-degree (longitude) line that belts the Earth, aka the equator.

Topographic maps show latitude and longitude as well as UTM grid lines. Known as UTM coordinates, the numbers index a specific point using a grid method. The survey datum used to arrive at the coordinates in this book is WGS84 (versus NAD27 or WGS83). Readers who own a GPS unit, whether handheld or in a vehicle, can enter the latitude and longitude or UTM coordinates provided on the last page of each hike. Just make sure your GPS unit is set to navigate using WGS84 datum, and you can navigate directly to the trailhead.

Most trailheads that begin in parking areas can be reached by car, but some hikes still require a short walk to reach the trailhead from a parking area. In those cases, a handheld unit is necessary to continue the GPS navigation process. That said, however, readers can easily access all trailheads in this book by using the directions, overview map, and trail map, which shows at least one major road leading into the area. But for those who enjoy using the latest GPS technology to navigate, the necessary data has been provided. A brief explanation of the UTM coordinates from Rosary Lakes (Hike 10) follows.

UTM zone (WGS84) 10T
Easting 578410
Northing 4827494
Latitude N43° 35.777'
Longitude W122° 1.714'

The UTM zone number 10 refers to one of the 60 vertical zones of the Universal Transverse Mercator projection. Each zone is 6 degrees wide. The UTM zone letter "T" refers to one of the 20 horizontal zones that span from 80 degrees south to 84 degrees north. The easting number 578410 indicates in meters how far east or west a point is from the central meridian of the zone. Increasing easting coordinates on a topo map or on your GPS screen indicate that you are moving east; decreasing easting coordinates indicate you are moving west. The northing number 4827494 references in meters how far you are from the equator. Above and below the equator, increasing northing coordinates indicate you are traveling north; decreasing northing coordinates indicate you are traveling south. To learn more about how to enhance your outdoor experiences with GPS technology, refer to *Outdoor Navigation with GPS* by Stephen Hinch.

THE HIKE PROFILE

In addition to maps, each hike contains a concise but informative narrative of the hike from beginning to end. This descriptive text is enhanced with at-a-glance ratings and information, GPS-based trailhead coordinates, and driving directions from a major road to the parking area most convenient to the trailhead.

At the top of the section for each hike is a box with pertinent information: quality of scenery, condition of trail, appropriateness for children, difficulty of hike, quality of solitude expected, hike distance, approximate time of hike, and outstanding highlights of the trip. The first five categories are rated using a five-star system. An example follows:

1 California Border to Observation Peak

SCENERY: ✰ ✰ ✰	HIKING TIME: *3 hours*
TRAIL CONDITION: ✰ ✰ ✰	MAP: *USFS* Applegate and West Ashland
CHILDREN: ✰ ✰	Ranger District
DIFFICULTY: ✰ ✰	OUTSTANDING FEATURES: *A geographical*
SOLITUDE: ✰ ✰ ✰ ✰	*curiosity, a quiet forest, and a sweeping, panoramic*
DISTANCE: *6 miles round-trip*	*viewpoint*

The three stars indicate the scenery is relatively picturesque. The two stars indicate it is a relatively easy hike (five stars for difficulty would be strenuous). The trail condition is good (one star would mean the trail is likely to be muddy, rocky, overgrown, or otherwise compromised). You can expect to encounter very few people on the trail (with one star you may well be elbowing your way up the trail). And the hike is possible but somewhat strenuous for able-bodied older children (a one-star rating would denote that only the most gung ho and physically fit children should go).

Distances given are absolute, but hiking times are estimated for an average hiking speed of 2 to 3 miles per hour, with time built in for pauses at overlooks and brief rests. Overnight hiking times account for the effort of carrying a backpack. All the other logistics you need (driving directions and permit and fee information) are grouped in a box with the GPS information at the end of each hike.

Following each box is a brief italicized description of the hike. A more detailed account follows that notes trail junctions, stream crossings, and trailside features along with their distance from the trailhead. Flip through the book, read the descriptions, and choose a hike that appeals to you.

Weather

THE HIKING SEASON ON OREGON'S PACIFIC CREST TRAIL is like a window that opens briefly and that you must dive through. To carry the analogy further, since the window opens (in July) and closes (in October), we have to be particularly careful, because July's lingering snow and swarming mosquitoes and October's worsening weather can make a trip something other than relaxing and fun. Because it is first and foremost a *crest* trail, the PCT is covered with snow from early November to at least late June, though some of these hikes, in some years, open up earlier. Still, even in July, on the higher and north-facing slopes, you'll potentially be walking on a few feet of snow. In a nutshell, think of July as settling down but having bugs, August as being filled with flowers and people, September as being pretty much perfect, and October as offering fall colors and your last chance to get up there. That's our PCT hiking season.

When planning a trip at these elevations, even in summer, expect anything from heat to snow. As a rule of thumb, the temperature decreases about 3 degrees for every 1,000 feet of elevation gained. Despite Oregon's reputation, there's very little rainfall, even in the mountains, in summer. As for temperatures, they can vary widely by location and elevation; what follows is a chart for Portland, which is near sea level. The Oregon PCT, on average, lies between 4,500 and 6,000 feet.

AVERAGE TEMPERATURE (FAHRENHEIT) BY MONTH

	JAN	FEB	MARCH	APRIL	MAY	JUNE
HIGH	45°	51°	56°	60°	67°	74°
LOW	34°	36°	38°	41°	47°	52°
	JULY	AUG	SEPT	OCT	NOV	DEC
HIGH	78°	80°	74°	64°	52°	45°
LOW	56°	56°	52°	44°	38°	34°

Water

How MUCH IS ENOUGH? Well, one simple physiological fact should persuade you to err on the side of excess when deciding how much water to pack: a hiker working hard in 90-degree heat needs approximately 10 quarts of fluid per day. That's 2.5 gallons—12 large water bottles or 16 small ones. In other words, pack one or two bottles even for short hikes.

Some hikers and backpackers hit the trail prepared to purify water found along the route. This method, while less dangerous than drinking it untreated, comes with risks. Purifiers with ceramic filters are the safest. Many hikers pack the slightly distasteful tetraglycine-hydroperiodide tablets to debug water (sold under the names Potable Aqua, Coughlan's, and others).

Probably the most common waterborne "bug" that hikers face is *Giardia,* which may not hit until up to four weeks after ingestion. Giardiasis will have you living in the bathroom, passing noxious rotten-egg gas, vomiting, and shivering with chills. Other parasites to worry about include *E. coli* and *cryptosporidium*, both of which are harder to kill than *Giardia.*

For most people, the pleasures of hiking make carrying water a relatively minor price to pay to remain healthy. If you're tempted to drink "found water," do so only if you understand the risks involved. Better yet, hydrate before your hike, carry (and drink) six ounces of water for every mile you plan to hike, and hydrate after the hike.

Clothing

IF YOU EVER HAVE A DAY TO KILL, simply find a dedicated PCT hiker and say to him or her, "What do you wear out there, and why?" Technological advances in materials and the recent lightweight revolution in clothing and equipment have turned an already gear-happy crowd into complete gear geeks and "ounce police." You don't have to be this way, but there are some basics you should stick to.

The first thing to remember is *layers, not cotton.* Wear layers. Don't wear cotton. Cotton, when wet, will make you more miserable than you'd be without it. Go instead with synthetics or wool (which, if you didn't know, is now way beyond its itchy reputation). The idea of layers is that as you hike and rest (getting warmer and cooler), and as the weather changes, you can be prepared for any combination of movement and conditions. Some kind of hat is highly recommended as well.

As for raingear, if you're reading this, either you're an Oregonian or have spent some time here, so I don't have to tell you that hiking around here without raingear is like going to a barbecue without an appetite: downright foolish. I recommend something light (think layers!) but as waterproof as you can stand it—by which I mean something that isn't rubber but also isn't so "breathable" that you wind up soaked after a few hours of rain.

A result of the lightweight revolution has been that many long-distance hikers can now be seen in running shoes or other light footwear. More power to them, I say. I still prefer the stiff soles of hiking boots, and I need their ankle support to avoid twists and sprains, but this doesn't mean you have to wear the leather Herman Munster jobs of 20 years ago. There are fantastic, fairly light, waterproof boots out there that won't break your budget; just make sure they don't give you blisters (or that you've prepared for such) before you take off on a 15-mile adventure.

The Ten Essentials

ONE OF THE FIRST RULES OF HIKING is to be prepared for anything. The simplest way to be prepared is to carry the Ten Essentials. In addition to carrying the items listed below, you need to know how to use them, especially navigation items. Always consider worst-case scenarios like getting lost, hiking back in the dark, breaking gear (for example, a broken hip strap on your pack or a water filter getting plugged), twisting an ankle, or encountering a brutal thunderstorm. The items listed below don't cost a lot of money, don't take up much room in a pack, and don't weigh much, but they might just save your life.

WATER: Durable bottles and a water treatment method like iodine or a filter

MAP: Preferably a topo map and a trail map with a route description

COMPASS: A high-quality compass

FIRST-AID KIT: A good-quality kit including first-aid instructions

KNIFE: A multitool device with pliers is best.

LIGHT: A flashlight or headlamp with extra bulbs and batteries

FIRE: Windproof matches or a lighter and fire starter

EXTRA FOOD: You should always have food in your pack when you've finished hiking.

EXTRA CLOTHES: Rain protection, warm layers, gloves, and a warm hat

SUN PROTECTION: Sunglasses, lip balm, sunblock, and a sun hat

First-Aid Kit

A TYPICAL FIRST-AID KIT may contain more items than you might think necessary. These are just the basics. Prepackaged kits in waterproof bags (Atwater Carey and Adventure Medical make a variety of kits) are available. Even though there are quite a few items listed here, they pack down into a small space:

Ace bandages or Spence joint wraps

Antibiotic ointment (Neosporin, polysporin, or a generic double- or triple-antibiotic cream)

Aspirin or acetaminophen

Band-Aids

Basic first-aid pamphlet (and the know-how to use it)

Benadryl or a generic equivalent diphenhydramine (in case of allergic reactions)

Butterfly wound-closure bandages

Epinephrine in a prefilled syringe (for people known to have severe allergic reactions to such things as bee stings)

Gauze (one roll and a half dozen 4- x 4-inch pads)

Hydrogen peroxide or iodine

Insect repellent

Irrigation syringe (to clean out wounds and prevent infection)

Matches or a pocket lighter

Moleskin or Spenco "Second Skin"

Sunscreen

Water-purification tablets

Whistle (it's more effective for signaling rescuers than your voice)

Hiking with Children

NO ONE IS TOO YOUNG FOR A HIKE. Be mindful though. Flat, short, and shaded trails are best with an infant. Toddlers who have not quite mastered walking can still tag along, riding on an adult's back in a child carrier. Use common sense to judge a child's capacity to hike a particular trail, and always expect that the child will tire quickly and need to be carried. A list of hikes suitable for children is provided on page xiii.

General Safety

TO SOME POTENTIAL MOUNTAIN ENTHUSIASTS, the deep woods seem inordinately dark and perilous. It is the fear of the unknown that causes this anxiety. No doubt, potentially dangerous situations can occur outdoors, but as long as you use sound judgment and prepare yourself before hitting the trail, you'll be much safer in the woods than in most urban areas of the country. It is better to look at a backcountry hike as a fascinating chance to discover the unknown rather than a chance for potential disaster. If you're new to the game, start out easy and find a person who knows what he or she is doing to help you out. These tips will make your trip safer and easier.

- ALWAYS CARRY FOOD AND WATER whether you are planning to go overnight or not. Food will give you energy, help keep you warm, and sustain you in an emergency until help arrives. You never know if you will have a stream nearby when you become thirsty. Bring potable water or treat water before drinking it from a stream. Boil or filter all found water before drinking it.

- STAY ON DESIGNATED TRAILS. Most hikers get lost when they leave the path. Even on the most clearly marked trails, there is usually a point where you have to stop and consider which way to go. If you become disoriented, don't panic. As soon as you think you may be off-track, stop, assess your current direction, and then retrace your steps to the point where you went awry. Using a map, a compass, and this book, and keeping in mind what you have passed thus far, reorient yourself, and trust your judgment on which way to proceed. If you become absolutely unsure of how to continue, return to your vehicle the way you came in. Should you become completely lost and have no idea how to return to the trailhead, remaining in place along the trail and waiting for help is most often the best option for adults and always the best option for children.

- BE ESPECIALLY CAREFUL WHEN CROSSING STREAMS. Whether you are fording a stream or crossing one on a log, make every step count. If you have any doubt about maintaining your balance on a foot log, go ahead and ford the stream instead. Or if the stream is too deep to ford, you could also sit down on a log and scoot across it. When fording a stream, use a trekking pole or stout stick for balance and face upstream as you cross. If a stream seems too deep to ford, turn back. Whatever is on the other side is not worth risking your life for.

- BE CAREFUL AT OVERLOOKS. While these areas may provide spectacular views, they are potentially hazardous. Stay back from the edge of outcrops, and be absolutely sure of your footing; a misstep can mean a nasty and possibly fatal fall.

- BEWARE: Standing dead trees and storm-damaged living trees pose a real hazard to hikers and tent campers. These trees may have loose or broken limbs that could fall at any time. When choosing a spot to rest or a backcountry campsite, look up.

- KNOW THE SYMPTOMS OF HYPOTHERMIA. Shivering and forgetfulness are the two most common indicators of this insidious killer. Hypothermia can occur at any elevation, even in the summer, especially when a hiker is wearing lightweight cotton clothing. If symptoms arise, get the victim shelter, hot liquids, and dry clothes or a dry sleeping bag.

- TAKE ALONG YOUR BRAIN. A cool, calculating mind is the single most important piece of equipment you'll ever need on the trail. Think before you act. Watch your step. Plan ahead. Avoiding accidents before they happen is the best recipe for a rewarding and relaxing hike.

- ASK QUESTIONS. National and state forest and park employees are there to help. It's a lot easier to get advice beforehand and thereby avoid a mishap. Use your head out there, and treat the place as if it were your own backyard—because it is.

Animal and Plant Hazards

MY BASIC THEORY IS THAT MOST PEOPLE WORRY TOO MUCH about stuff in the woods. There's not an animal on the Oregon PCT that wants to cause you trouble, unless you count ticks and mosquitoes. And as for plants, you'll hardly ever see poison oak on a hike in this book. So make a plan for ticks based on this information, pick a time when skeeters won't be a problem, and then hope you'll be lucky enough to see something like a bear or coyote. And stop worrying!

TICKS

On the Oregon PCT, you have a slight chance of encountering ticks in the Siskiyous and virtually no chance of encountering them anywhere else this book covers. Still, let's cover the basics: Ticks like to hang out in the brush that grows along trails. Their numbers explode in hot summer months, but you should be tick-aware during all months of the year. Ticks, which are arthropods and not insects, need a host to feast on to reproduce. The ticks that light onto you while you're hiking will be very small, sometimes so tiny that you won't be able to spot them.

They're primarily of two varieties, deer ticks and dog ticks; both need a few hours of actual attachment before they can transmit any disease they may harbor (Lyme disease or Rocky Mountain spotted fever, for instance). Ticks may settle in shoes, socks, and hats and may take several hours to latch on to skin. The best strategy is to visually check every half hour or so while hiking, do a thorough check before you get in the car, and then, when you take a post-hike shower, do an even more thorough check of your entire body. Ticks that haven't attached are easily removed but not easily killed. If you pick off a tick in the woods, just toss it aside. If you find one on your body at home, dispatch it and then send it down the toilet. For ticks that have embedded, removal with tweezers is best.

SNAKES

There certainly are rattlesnakes in Oregon, but they're not 5,000 feet up in the mountains, and they aren't west of the Cascades, either. If you see a snake on any of these hikes, it will be a harmless and terrified garter snake, getting away from you as fast as it can.

OTHER CRITTERS

I hear there are black bears in Oregon, but in ten years of hiking, I've never seen one, except on the Rogue River. And everybody I know who has seen one has reported the bears doing the same thing: running the heck away. Same thing goes for all big cats, like mountain lions and bobcats, as well as elk—not that you'd be worried about elk. Especially if you're quiet and it's early or late in the day, you might see the occasional coyote or deer, and at some point you will have the heart-stopping experience of scaring up a trailside grouse. Basically, the only animals you need to worry about are the ones on two legs.

Poison Ivy, Oak, and Sumac

In Oregon, poison ivy, oak, and sumac generally don't exist above 3,000 feet—which is to say they shouldn't be a problem in the areas covered by this book. Still, some of the lower-elevation hikes, especially down south, might have them, so we'll go with the standard advice here. Avoiding contact with these plants is the most effective way to prevent the painful, itchy rashes their oils can cause.

Poison ivy ranges from a thick, tree-hugging vine to a shaded ground cover, three leaflets to a leaf; poison oak occurs as either a vine or a shrub, with three leaflets as well; and poison sumac flourishes in swampland, with each leaf having 7 to 13 leaflets. Urushiol, the oil in the sap of these plants, is responsible for the rash. Usually within 12 to 14 hours of exposure (but sometimes much later), you'll see raised lines and/or blisters and experience a terrible itch.

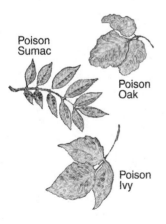

Poison Sumac

Poison Oak

Poison Ivy

Refrain from scratching because bacteria under your fingernails can cause infection. Wash and dry the rash thoroughly, applying a calamine lotion or other product to help dry the rash. Once you've washed the urushiol off your skin, the rash will not spread, but it may take a few days for all the affected areas to break out. If itching or blistering is severe, seek medical attention. Remember that oil-contaminated clothes, pets, or hiking gear can easily cause an irritating rash on you or someone else. Wash not only any exposed parts of your body but also clothes, gear, and pets.

MOSQUITOES

Oregon is known for rain, right? And the Cascades get a lot of snow? And when the snow melts, there's a lot of water around, right? And where do mosquitoes live? That's right, the Cascades. July or anytime right after the snow has melted is the time of the mosquito in the Oregon mountains. If you're doing any of these hikes then, think seriously about wearing long sleeves and bringing repellent and a tent. This is especially true of any high-elevation hike that visits a lake (Sky Lakes, for example).

Although it's not a common occurrence, individuals can become infected with the West Nile virus by being bitten by an infected mosquito. Culex mosquitoes, the primary varieties that can transmit West Nile virus to humans, thrive in urban rather than natural areas. They lay their eggs in stagnant water and can breed in any standing water that remains for more than five days. Most people infected with West Nile virus have no symptoms of illness, but some may become ill, usually 3 to 15 days after being bitten.

Tips for Enjoying the PCT in Oregon

- WHEN YOU'VE READ A DSCRIPTION AND ARE READY TO HIT THE TRAIL, it's best to make sure you can go. Is the road open? Is the trail washed out? Is there a fire? Call the the local national forest ranger district (see contact information in Appendix B, page 188) before leaving home.

- DON'T LET A HIKE'S LISTED DISTANCE OR ITS ELEVATION PROFILE DISCOURAGE YOU from trying it. In almost all cases, there are fine attractions along the way, meaning you don't have to deal with that part of the profile that looks like a parking cone, or you don't actually have to put in, say, 20-plus miles to enjoy the Sky Lakes Wilderness.

- TAKE YOUR TIME ALONG THE TRAILS. Pace yourself. The forest is filled with wonders both big and small. Don't rush past a tiny salamander to get to that overlook. Stop and smell the wildflowers. Peer into a clear mountain stream for brook trout. Don't miss the trees for the forest. Shorter hikes allow you to stop and linger more than long hikes. Something about heading out on a 10-mile trek naturally pushes you to speed up. That said, take close notice of the elevation maps that accompany each hike. If you see many ups and downs over large altitude changes, you'll obviously need more time. Inevitably, you'll finish some hikes long before or after what is suggested. Nevertheless, leave yourself plenty of time for those moments when you simply feel like stopping and taking it all in.

- HERE'S ANOTHER THING TO TRY: KEEP YOUR HEAD UP. No, I don't mean "don't get discouraged"; I mean quit looking at the trail all the time. Sometimes, when I lead a hike, I tell people at the trailhead to take a good look at their boots and then at the ground, and then I ask them to take my word for it that these things won't change. The views above, however, change constantly, and with a little practice you'll find you can trust your feet a lot more than you realized to get you over rocks and roots.

- WE CAN'T ALWAYS SCHEDULE OUR FREE TIME WHEN WE WANT, but try to hike during the week and avoid the weekends if possible. Trails that are packed on Saturday and Sunday are often clear during the week. If you are hiking on a busy day, go early in the morning; it'll enhance your chances of seeing wildlife. The trails really clear out during rainy times, but don't hike during a thunderstorm.

Backcountry Advice

IN ALL BUT A FEW CASES for the trails covered in this book, a permit is not required before entering the backcountry to camp. However, you should practice low-impact camping. Adhere to the adages "Pack it in; pack it out" and "Take only pictures; leave only footprints." Practice "Leave no trace" camping ethics while in the backcountry.

Open fires are often not permitted, especially near lakes, in high-use areas and during dry times when the Forest Service may

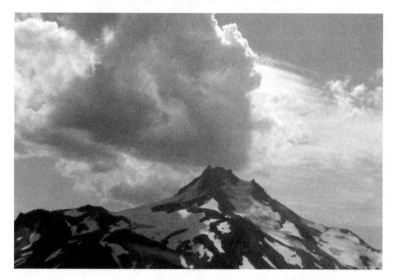

Mount Jefferson from the top of Park Butte, which can be reached from Hike 18 or 19

issue a fire ban. Backpacking stoves are strongly encouraged. You might want to hang your food out of the reach of bears and other animals to minimize human impact on wildlife and avoid their introduction to and dependence on human food. Wildlife learns to associate backpacks and backpackers with easy food sources, thereby influencing their behavior.

Bring about 40 feet of thin but sturdy rope to properly secure your food. Ideally, you should throw your rope over a stout limb that extends ten or more feet above ground. Make sure it hangs at least five feet away from the tree trunk.

Bury solid human waste in a hole at least three inches deep and at least 200 feet away from trails and water sources; a trowel is basic backpacking equipment. Pack out all toilet paper.

Following the above guidelines will increase your chances for a pleasant, safe, and low-impact interaction with nature. The suggestions are intended to enhance your experience of the Cascade Mountains' flora and fauna. Forest regulations can change over time; contact Forest Service ranger stations to confirm the status of any regulations before you enter the backcountry.

Trail Etiquette

WHETHER YOU'RE ON A TRAIL IN A CITY, county, state, or national park, always remember that great care and resources (from nature as well as from your tax dollars) have gone into creating these trails. Treat the trail, wildlife, and your fellow hikers with respect.

- HIKE ON OPEN TRAILS ONLY. Respect trail and road closures (ask if you are not sure), avoid possible trespassing on private land, and obtain all permits and authorization as required. Also, leave gates as you found them or as marked.

- LEAVE ONLY FOOTPRINTS. Be sensitive to the ground beneath you. Stay on the existing trail and don't blaze new ones. Be sure to pack out what you pack in. No one likes to see the trash someone else has left behind.

- NEVER SPOOK ANIMALS. An unannounced approach, a sudden movement, or a loud noise startles most animals. A surprised animal can be dangerous to you, others, and itself. Give them plenty of space. Remember that you're the visitor.

- PLAN AHEAD. Know your equipment, your ability, and the area in which you are hiking—and prepare accordingly. Be self-sufficient at all times; carry the supplies necessary to adapt to changes in weather or other conditions. A well-executed trip will satisfy you and others.

- BE COURTEOUS TO OTHER HIKERS, BIKERS, AND EQUESTRIANS you encounter on the trails.

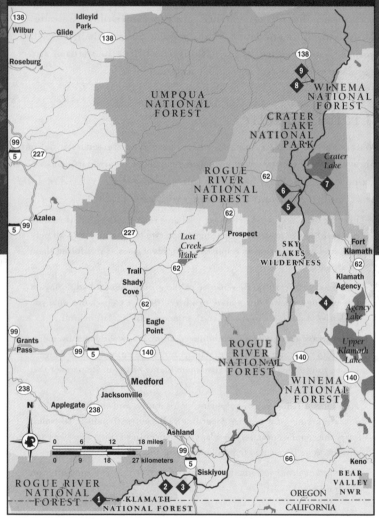

1

SOUTH

CALIFORNIA BORDER TO
MOUNT THIELSEN

1   California Border to Observation Peak (*page 20*)

2   Grouse Gap to Siskiyou Peak (*page 25*)

3   OR 99 to Pilot Rock (*page 30*)

4   Sky Lakes Wilderness (*page 36*)

5   OR 62 to Pumice Flat (*page 42*)

6   OR 62 to Crater Lake Rim (*page 47*)

7   Crater Lake Rim (*page 52*)

8   Mount Thielsen Loop (*page 58*)

9   Tipsoo Peak and Maidu Lake (*page 64*)

1 California Border to Observation Peak

> SCENERY: ☘ ☘ ☘
> TRAIL CONDITION: ☘ ☘ ☘
> CHILDREN: ☘ ☘
> DIFFICULTY: ☘ ☘
> SOLITUDE: ☘ ☘ ☘ ☘
> DISTANCE: 6 miles round-trip
>
> HIKING TIME: 3 hours
> MAP: USFS Applegate and West Ashland Ranger District
> OUTSTANDING FEATURES: A geographical curiosity, a quiet forest, and a sweeping, panoramic viewpoint

If you ever wanted to say you hiked from one state to another, here's your chance. Enter Oregon the way northbound Pacific Crest Trail thru-hikers do, and then climb the state's first peak for a lovely viewpoint—all without working too hard at all.

🚶 Being something of a map geek, I had to tell people how to hike to the Oregon–California border. It's less than a quarter mile from a road, but that isn't really the point of this hike. Observation Peak is the point. And for the record, I would have included the walk from Oregon to Washington as well, but it's across the narrow Bridge of the Gods at Cascade Locks, which has lots of traffic and no walkway. So this is your only chance for a border hike in this book.

From the road, start south (right, as you drove up) through meadows and thin forest, for a quarter mile down to a register at the border. You can join the hundreds of others who have taken their pictures next to the "Oregon" and "California" signs on a tree, enjoy the views south into the Golden State's Donomore Meadows, and read the exuberant comments of the thru-hikers who have tromped some 1,600 miles just to get through one state. Most of them arrive here around mid-August, having started at the Mexico–California border around May 1. But their speeds vary greatly: On one September hike here, I encountered a northbounder who said he liked to "sleep late, nap after lunch, and have a good time." At the other

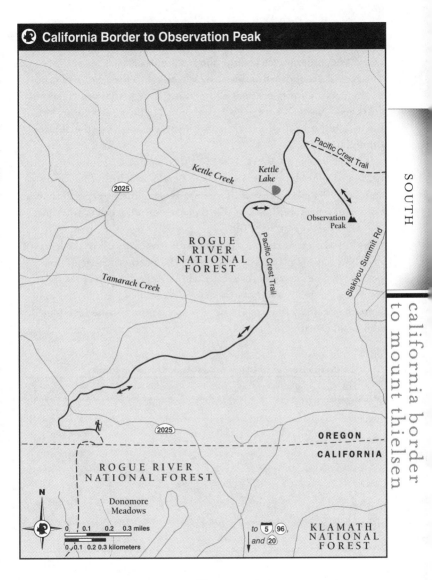

Pacific Crest Trail

Kettle Creek

Kettle Lake

2025

Observation Peak

SOUTH

Siskiyou Summit Rd

ROGUE RIVER NATIONAL FOREST

Pacific Crest Trail

Tamarack Creek

2025

OREGON

CALIFORNIA

N

ROGUE RIVER NATIONAL FOREST

Donomore Meadows

0   0.1   0.2   0.3 miles

0   0.1   0.2   0.3 kilometers

to 5 96, and 20

KLAMATH NATIONAL FOREST

california border to mount thielsen

extreme, I met a man at Washington's Snoqualmie Pass one August 30, then saw that he had signed this register on August 4. That's about 700 miles in 26 days, or about 27 miles a day!

Now sufficiently humbled, trek back up to the road and cross it, then start a long, gradual climb along a ridge that was clear-cut years ago. Now it's covered with chaparral, whose red blooms are a favorite of hummingbirds. Up ahead you can see your destination, Observation Peak.

When you've gone 2.3 miles, you'll come upon a sunny ridge that is the west shoulder of the peak. From here, you'll be in the forest for a bit and even cross a few small springs. It gets a little steeper at times, but it's never severe. Look for Kettle Lake down the hill to your left.

Half a mile past that little ridge, pop back into the open, with views to your left of rolling, forested hills stretching off to the horizon. Next, at a big rock pile, encounter the northern ridge of the peak, with fine views out toward Dutchman's Peak and its lookout. According to the book *Oregon Geographical Names,* this peak got its name from the death by freezing in the 1870s of a miner named Hensley . . . who was German. Go figure.

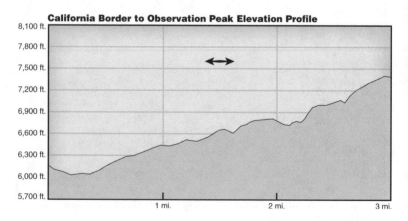

California Border to Observation Peak Elevation Profile

22

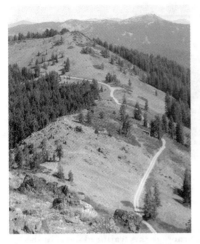

The trail now swings southeast and starts a traverse of the north side of Observation Peak, but you step off the trail just before it disappears into the woods, which are often filled with snow well into July. A short climb of 50 feet will put you on the ridgeline, which you then follow cross-country past several false summits to the real one, which is marked by a pile of rocks with a wood stake in it.

The PCT parallels FS 20 along the Siskiyou spine, seen from Observation Peak.

From the broad and grassy summit, which is a little more than 7,300 feet in elevation, you can make out FS 20 heading east toward Interstate 5 (the PCT stays very close to it all the way there), and off to the northeast, Mount McLoughlin. Farther east is Pilot Rock, the next big PCT attraction to the north and Hike 3 (page 30) in this book. Looking south, you'll see Mount Shasta, with the Marble Mountains to its right. And finally, in a red can among the rocks, there's a summit register with (when I was there) entries going back to October 20, 1992. The can was also, when I opened it, filled with hundreds of ladybugs.

A mildly interesting note about this summit is that it has two benchmarks labeled USC&GS, which stands for US Coast and Geodetic Survey, a government agency that was founded in 1807 by Thomas Jefferson but hasn't existed under that name since 1970.

You can cut some distance off your return trip by going cross-country to the west. You can't miss the trail down there, but since the going is steep and brushy in spots, I don't recommend it.

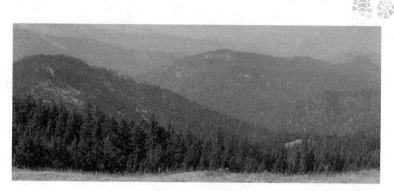

Looking north into the Siskiyous, from Observation Peak

DIRECTIONS The most direct route to this trailhead starts in the town of Jacksonville. From there, take OR 238 southwest for 7 miles to Ruch, and then take Upper Applegate Rd. south for 9 miles to FS 20, which branches left (east). Follow FS 20 (which eventually becomes gravel) for 14.5 miles to Silver Fork Gap, and turn southeast (downhill) on FS 2025, which is signed for Donomore Meadows. From there, it's 4.1 miles to the saddle where the PCT crosses the road.

You can also access this area from I-5 to the east, which would make sense only if you were already in the Mount Ashland area or doing our Pilot Rock (Hike 3, page 30) or Siskiyou Peak hikes (Hike 2, page 25). From I-5, follow FS 20 (the Mount Ashland Rd.) for 27 miles to Silver Fork Gap. Only the first 9 of these miles are paved, and some of the miles west of Meridian Overlook are quite rough.

PERMIT None

GPS Trailhead Coordinates	1 California Border to Observation Peak
UTM Zone (WGS84)	10T
Easting	507280
Northing	465031
Latitude	N42° 0.292'
Longitude	W122° 54.725'

2 Grouse Gap to Siskiyou Peak

SCENERY: ♦ ♦ ♦ ♦	HIKING TIME: *2½ hours*
TRAIL CONDITION: ♦ ♦ ♦	MAP: *USFS* Applegate and West Ashland
CHILDREN: ♦ ♦ ♦ ♦	Ranger District
DIFFICULTY: ♦ ♦ ♦	OUTSTANDING FEATURES: *A shelter to camp*
SOLITUDE: ♦ ♦ ♦ ♦	*or picnic in; interesting forest, flower-filled bowls;*
DISTANCE: *5.2 miles round-trip*	*and a wide open mountain viewpoint*

Take a stroll up to, and then along, the spine of the Siskiyou Mountains, from a big shelter to one of the range's highest peaks. You'll see big trees, interesting rock formations, wild-flowers galore, and a view that stretches for miles and miles.

This Siskiyou section of the Pacific Crest Trail does something fairly interesting: It runs generally east and west, which might seem odd for a trail that goes from Mexico to Canada. It does so because if the trail were to go due north from the Mount Shasta area of far northern California to the area around Pilot Rock, east of here, it would cover many dry, difficult miles. In fact, before the trail was officially completed, this latter path was the route hikers took. To avoid this, the trail was built in the 1970s to swing way to the west in California, cross into Oregon, and here swing way back to the east, following the spine of the Siskiyous.

That's why, when you start walking "south" on the PCT from Grouse Gap, you're actually walking to the west, and not far "north" of you, the trail swings back to the southeast. Whichever way you're headed, start by walking down the road to the Grouse Gap Shelter, which is especially popular with winter recreationists who follow FS 20 into the mountains. At the shelter, you'll find a restroom, picnic tables, a huge fire pit, and a fence to keep the cows out. You can also camp here, as many PCT hikers do. I spent a night in the shelter once and heard coyotes howling and two owls hooting at each other.

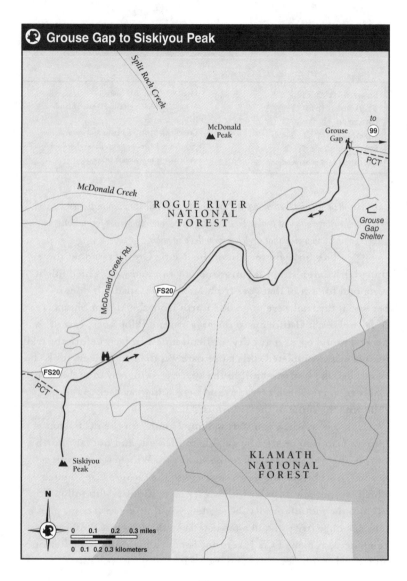

Grouse Gap to Siskiyou Peak

Split Rock Creek

McDonald Peak

Grouse Gap

to 99

PCT

McDonald Creek

ROGUE RIVER NATIONAL FOREST

Grouse Gap Shelter

McDonald Creek Rd.

FS20

FS20

PCT

Siskiyou Peak

KLAMATH NATIONAL FOREST

N

0   0.1   0.2   0.3 miles

0   0.1 0.2 0.3 kilometers

Back at the road, look for the PCT headed west and uphill, just on the south side of FS 20. Start in the open for 0.2 mile, then climb into an impressive hemlock forest filled with snags and blow-downs, many of them covered with an intensely bright green moss. The rocky ridge up ahead is your next destination.

A little less than a mile out, you reach a section of forest that's interesting because there's nothing else growing in it; it's just bare, sandy ground and trees. As you get up toward the ridge, look left for Mount Ashland with a big white ball (a weather radar station) on its summit. Below it and to the right, look for Pilot Rock, which the PCT visits in Hike 3 (page 30) of this book. At 0.9 mile, the trail gets steeper and makes a switchback to the right, with interesting rock formations above you marking the ridgetop.

When you reach the saddle, you'll see the trail ahead of you, traversing the top of a large bowl, which, in summer and early fall, is filled with flowers. Also visible are two humps on the ridge; the one on the left is Siskiyou Peak. You'll also see that you're essentially back at FS 20, and in fact if you walk up to it, you'll get a view all the way to spiny Mount Thielsen, some 80 miles northeast as the crow flies—and about 150 miles on the PCT.

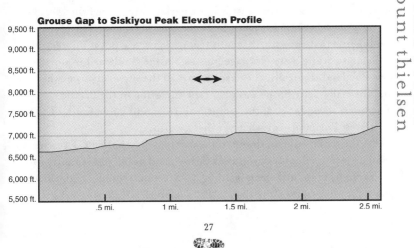

Grouse Gap to Siskiyou Peak Elevation Profile

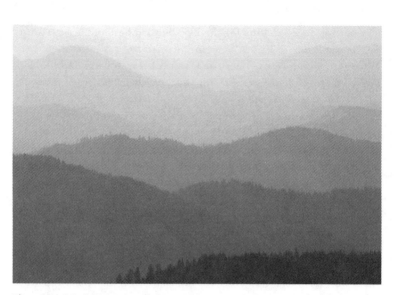

The ridges of the Siskiyous from Siskiyou Peak

Drop over the ridge into the south-facing bowl, and start gradually downhill, now going west. Toward the far end of the bowl, you almost touch FS 20 again, just below a parking area called the Meridian Overlook because it's near the Willamette Meridian. The Meridian is a line that runs north-south from a reference point located in Willamette Stone State Heritage Site on Skyline Boulevard in northwest Portland. Basically, they had to start all the surveying somewhere, and the Willamette Stone was where the surveying in the Pacific Northwest started. So, at this point, you're standing due south of northwest Portland—for whatever that's worth.

A third of a mile southwest of the overlook, when the PCT reaches a saddle just north of Siskiyou Peak, leave it and head cross-country to the summit. It's a little steep (gaining 400 feet in 0.3 mile) and, since you're heading up to more than 7,000 feet in elevation, you may get winded. But the view from the top is worth it, and there's even a summit register for you to sign. This is an excellent place to watch a sunset, by the way, especially if you park a car at the Meridian Overlook.

DIRECTIONS From Ashland, go 12 miles south on I-5, and take Exit 6 for Mount Ashland. This exit puts you on OR 99, which you follow south for 1 mile, still following signs for Mount Ashland. Turn right (west) onto paved Mount Ashland Rd., which turns into FS 20.

In 9 miles, you reach the Mount Ashland Ski Area, and 0.2 mile later leave the pavement. Stay right at a junction in 0.1 mile, and 2.4 miles later you reach Grouse Gap. Park here, on the right side of the road, or turn left and go 0.3 mile to Grouse Gap Shelter, where there's more parking and a restroom.

PERMITS None

GPS Trailhead Coordinates	2 Grouse Gap to Siskiyou Peak
UTM Zone (WGS84)	10T
Easting	521552
Northing	4658886
Latitude	N42° 4.905'
Longitude	W122° 44.366'

3 OR 99 to Pilot Rock

SCENERY: 🐾 🐾 🐾	MAP: *USFS East Ashland Ranger District*
TRAIL CONDITION: 🐾 🐾 🐾	HIKING TIME: *5 hours*
CHILDREN: 🐾 🐾 🐾	OUTSTANDING FEATURES: *Rolling hills, open*
DIFFICULTY: 🐾 🐾	*grasslands, wildflowers, wide views, solitude, and*
SOLITUDE: 🐾 🐾 🐾 🐾	*some optional rock climbing*
DISTANCE: *9.2 miles round-trip*	

Take a little trip through cowboy country—literally. This hike wanders through former log-ging and grazing lands that are being restored to their natural state. You'll get some nice viewpoints that stretch into California, and you can visit a southern Oregon landmark.

🚶🚶 Among PCT hikers, this section of the trail is, shall we say, widely disrespected. The quasi-official guidebook for thru-hikers calls it "the driest, least scenic section" in Oregon and Washington, adding that it "will certainly be shunned by many" other than "long-distance hikers passing through to a more scenic destination."

Heed not such discouraging words. I happen to like the walk up to Pilot Rock for its unique character, rolling-hills cowboy feel, and solitude. And if you feel like doing a little climbing, there's a nice view as well.

If you want to skip the bulk of this hike, it's possible to drive to within a mile of Pilot Rock's summit. My directions below are to the lower trailhead. To reach the upper trailhead (which you will also hike to by following these hiking directions, making a shuttle possible), drive 0.6 mile past the lower trailhead on OR 99, and turn left (east) on Pilot Rock Road. This bumpy track will lead you 2 miles to a big turnout area, from which you need to stay uphill on the second road from the left. It's another bumpy mile up to the trailhead at the end of the road.

But let's do the whole walk instead. Starting from your trailhead on OR 99, dip down briefly to cross a gully, and then wind your way

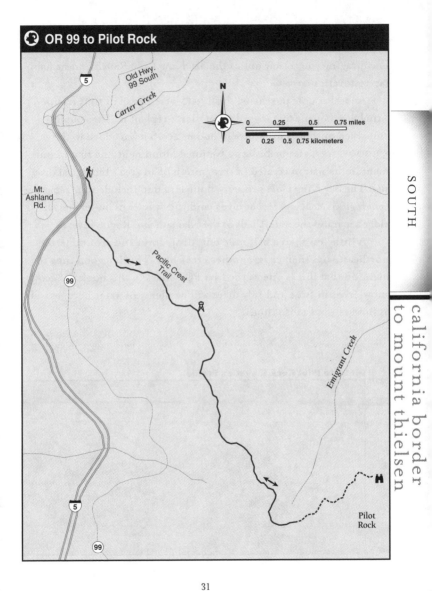

N

| 0 | 0.25 | 0.5 | 0.75 miles |
| 0 | 0.25 | 0.5 | 0.75 kilometers |

Old Hwy. 99 South

Carter Creek

Mt. Ashland Rd.

99

Pacific Crest Trail

Emigrant Creek

Pilot Rock

SOUTH

california border to mount thielsen

up through open grasslands. Cross over a little creek (probably dry by late summer) at 0.3 mile, and you will see the first of many signs encouraging you to stay out of the Sky King Cole Ranch and its habitat-restoration area.

A local couple purchased this 1,300-acre parcel in 1991 from a timber company that logged it but didn't replant it. The couple embarked on a plan to restore it, and in 2006 it was added to the 53,000-acre Cascade-Siskiyou National Monument, the first monument in the nation created in recognition of an area's biological diversity. The Sky King Cole property alone is said to include four separate eco-regions, 200 species of birds, and 100 species of butterflies. Its ridge separates the watersheds of the Klamath and Rogue Rivers.

A little less than a half mile out, drop down and around to the northeast, and then cross another creek bed. This is a good time to mention that this is one of the first PCT hikes in this book to become snow-free; in June and July there will be plenty of water here, as well as flowers—and mosquitoes.

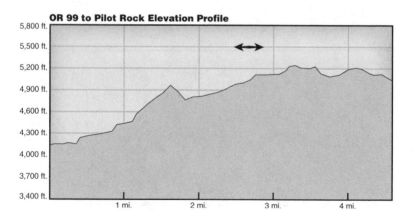

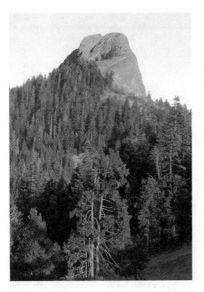

Pilot Rock from a viewpoint on the PCT

About 0.6 mile out, cross a footbridge and an old road, then climb to the south. Look for views of Mount Ashland across Interstate 5, and also (just past a boardwalk at 0.8 mile) a tremendous tree on your right, with a swooping canopy that touches the ground below you to the left.

After 1.4 miles, switchback to the left at a piece of metal pipe in the ground, and begin a gradual climb to the east that tops out in a flat meadow. A few minutes later, pass through a gate with a Bureau of Land Management sign (be sure to close the gate behind you), and see a communication tower just ahead. If that's not appealing to you, look right for more nice views back to the Siskiyou Range and Mount Ashland.

Round the top of a ridge at 1.8 miles, cross over a little piece of boardwalk that seems to serve no purpose whatsoever, and then commence another flat section bending to the west with a nice view north. You're heading for the end of that ridge you see. In this section, right at 2 miles, there's a turn that could be easy to miss. Look for a stump on your left with four trail markers and, just past that, a stake marking a left turn.

Stroll downhill now, gaining your first view of Pilot Rock. You're walking almost due south, even though you're technically northbound on the PCT. That's because the trail here is coming out

33

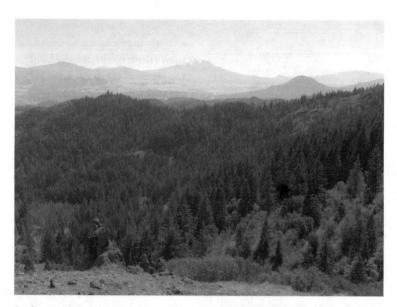

Looking south at California's Mount Shasta from the PCT near Pilot Rock

of a long eastward swing through the Siskiyous. The final turn north, for Canada, is just before the upper trailhead on this hike.

At 2.2 miles, you come to an intersection where the trail descends just east of a road, and then enjoy a nice ridgetop walk to another, major road crossing. The trail continues across the main road and between two others headed south, and then it climbs gradually to a long, open ridge with views of ever-closer Pilot Rock. After a mile and a half of this, you'll drop down to yet another road, this time at the upper trailhead parking area.

Continue across the lot on the PCT, which is now very wide because of all the folks coming up to climb Pilot Rock. In 0.2 mile, you have to make a decision: If you want to climb the rock itself, take the wider trail heading up and to the right. I have not done this route, since every time I've been up here the weather has been unpleasant, so I cannot comment on it directly. However, other hikers and a Forest Service ranger inform me that it's straightforward, hands-and-feet rock scrambling that doesn't require a rope.

The PCT stays left of the summit trail and in 100 yards arrives at a wonderful wooden backpack rest. I have seen a journal in it with fun thru-hiker comments. Next, pass several interesting rock formations, one of which has a view left to Mount McLoughlin.

Finally, a total of 4.6 miles out, you'll come to a fine viewpoint on a shoulder of Pilot Rock's ridge. Mount Shasta is off to the south, Pilot Rock looms to your right, and there's a volcanic plug on the trail right in front of you. Volcanic or not, it makes a fine place to sit down, have a snack, and take it all in.

DIRECTIONS From Ashland, go south on I-5 for 12 miles, and take Exit 6 for Mount Ashland. This exit puts you on OR 99, which you follow south for 1.4 miles to a gravel parking area on the left shoulder. There's no official sign here, but in various years the spot has been marked by a ribbon on a tree, a rock cairn, and a makeshift PCT sign. (See text for directions to the upper trailhead and a shorter hiking option.)

PERMITS None

GPS Trailhead Coordinates	3 OR 99 to Pilot Rock
UTM Zone (WGS84)	10T
Easting	532991
Northing	4657348
Latitude	N42° 4.050'
Longitude	W122° 36.073'

4 Sky Lakes Wilderness

SCENERY: 🐾 🐾 🐾 🐾	HIKING TIME: *3 days*
TRAIL CONDITION: 🐾 🐾 🐾	MAP: *USFS* Sky Lakes Wilderness
CHILDREN: 🐾 🐾	OUTSTANDING FEATURES: *A series of high-*
DIFFICULTY: 🐾 🐾 🐾	*altitude lakes, mountain views, and a dramatic*
SOLITUDE: 🐾 🐾	*ridgeline walk*
DISTANCE: *23.8 miles*	

Officially, the Pacific Crest Trail skips the best parts of Sky Lakes Wilderness. To limit impact on the lakes, it runs along a high ridge away from all water. But most people skip that part and visit the lakes; I suggest you do both. **Warning:** *Do not go to the Sky Lakes in July or early August. The mosquitoes will absolutely ruin your trip. Trust me, I know.*

🏃🏃 Several trails access this wilderness, but what I am suggest-ing here is the easiest way in. That's because the hike in is a little more than 5 miles and gains all of 200 feet in elevation. From there, I suggest spending two nights with a long day hike in the middle, or perhaps even a third night to explore around the lake basin, going off-trail and maybe looking for some killer fishing.

Start at the Cold Spring Trailhead, where there's a shelter to spend the night but signs say the water isn't fit for drinking. Anyway, if you make it here by midday, you'll have plenty of time to find good camping in the woods. This is easy and pleasant walking, through an old forest where the biggest and most interesting trees are mountain hemlocks. In a little less than a mile you pass the South Rock Creek Trail (#3709), and then at 2.7 miles you join the Sky Lakes Trail (#3762), which comes in from the left.

Stick with the Sky Lakes Trail as it keeps rolling along, over tiny rises on a trail made wide by horses. You see huckleberries, some impressive trail building in a boulder field, and a little more than 3 miles out pass the Heavenly Twin Lakes, where all the campsites are

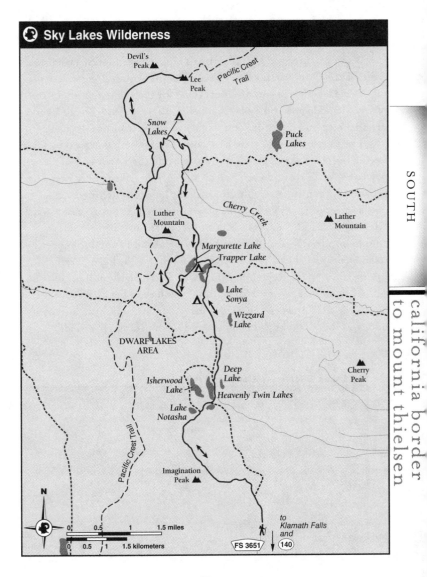

Devil's
Peak ▲▲

▲▲ Lee
Peak

Pacific Crest
Trail

Snow
Lakes

△

Puck
Lakes

Luther
Mountain
▲

Cherry Creek

▲ Lather
Mountain

Margurette Lake
Trapper Lake
△

● Lake
Sonya

△

Wizzard
Lake

DWARF LAKES
AREA

Deep
Lake

Cherry
Peak ▲

Isherwood
Lake

Heavenly Twin Lakes

Lake
Notasha

Pacific Crest Trail

Imagination
Peak ▲▲

N

0   0.5   1   1.5 miles

0   0.5   1   1.5 kilometers

to
Klamath Falls
and
140

FS 3651

closed for restoration. Fear not, for you're only 2 more easy miles from the main lake area and a bounty of campsites.

When you arrive at big, beautiful Trapper Lake (and see Cherry Creek Trail #3708 on the right), start looking around for camping. Some lakeshores are off-limits (look for the signs), but there are plenty of good spots. Some lakes are even off-trail. Just consult a good, detailed map and go for it. You might even get a trout for dinner.

The next morning, take the Divide Trail, which you find by following the Sky Lakes Trail as it wraps around the north end of Trapper Lake. Walk around even bigger Margurette Lake, where camping is banned, then the trail climbs gradually before switching back to pass a series of rocky viewpoints down into the lake basin, east toward Klamath Lake, and south to Mount McLoughlin. The scramble a couple hundred feet up Luther Mountain ahead of you looks pretty straightforward. Finally, 2.6 miles up from the Sky Lakes Trail, intersect the PCT. Remember the PCT? Turn right on it.

After all that lake and forest time, you'll see a big difference up here. The PCT traverses this ridge for 3.5 miles, with little bumps here and there and big views all around. In midsummer you also

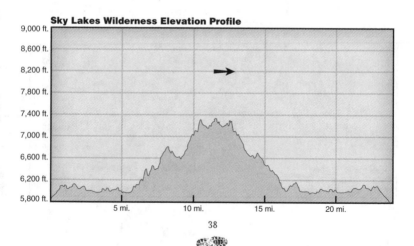

38

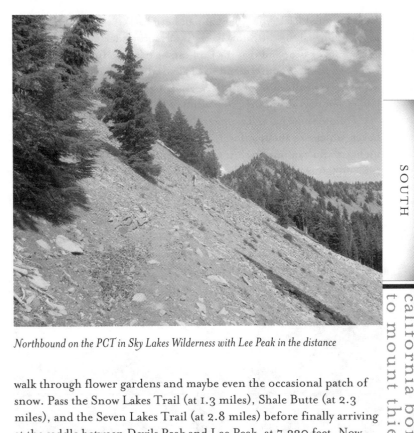

Northbound on the PCT in Sky Lakes Wilderness with Lee Peak in the distance

walk through flower gardens and maybe even the occasional patch of snow. Pass the Snow Lakes Trail (at 1.3 miles), Shale Butte (at 2.3 miles), and the Seven Lakes Trail (at 2.8 miles) before finally arriving at the saddle between Devils Peak and Lee Peak, at 7,320 feet. Now the view stretches from Mount McLoughlin in the south (and maybe even Mount Shasta if it's clear) to the peaks around Crater Lake, and beyond to pointy Mount Thielsen and the Three Sisters. In PCT miles, you're looking at a distance of well more than 100 miles.

Heading north, as you can see, you would drop down quite a slope, which until late July will have snow on it—lots of fun with a full backpack. But since there's not much to see between here and Crater

Lake National Park, you might as well head back. You could make a loop of it by taking the Snow Lakes Trail; just understand that would add a mile or two, and that the trail can be tricky to find. Basically, as you drop off the southern end of Shale Butte you'll hit a flat stretch with a sparse collection of small trees. The trail is in there, on the left; if you start dropping down again, you missed it.

Follow Snow Lakes Trail down 0.2 mile to the Upper Snow Lakes, which are about as lovely a place to spend some time (or a night) as you can imagine. At one campsite, somebody even made some furniture out of the flat stones. Beyond those lakes, your trail stays fairly flat for a half mile before the bottom drops out and you lose 700 feet in a little more than a mile down to the Nannie Creek Trail (#3707). This is also the northern end of the Sky Lakes Trail.

Trapper and Margurette Lakes, seen from Luther Mountain

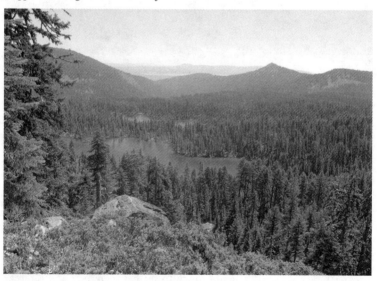

If you have a camp back among the lakes, that's your route home for the night. It's 2 easy miles from here to Margurette Lake.

And for the record, I officially don't know anything about feisty, 10- to 12-inch brook trout in any of these lakes, especially the bigger ones like . . . well, as I said, I'm not reporting any such thing. You didn't hear it from me.

DIRECTIONS From Klamath Falls, follow OR 140 for 22 miles west, and turn right onto FS 3651, which is signed for Cold Spring Trailhead. Follow this gravel road 11 miles to the trailhead at the end. If you're coming from Medford, this (left) turn is 41 miles east of OR 62 on the north end of town.

PERMITS A Northwest Forest Pass is required.

GPS Trailhead Coordinates	4 Sky Lakes Wilderness
UTM Zone (WGS84)	10T
Easting	567283
Northing	4710363
Latitude	N42° 32.5640'
Longitude	W122° 10.8350'

5 OR 62 to Pumice Flat

SCENERY: ☆ ☆	DISTANCE: *Up to 15 miles*
TRAIL CONDITION: ☆ ☆ ☆	HIKING TIME: *7 hours*
CHILDREN: ☆ ☆ ☆	MAP: Crater Lake National Park
DIFFICULTY: ☆	OUTSTANDING FEATURES: *Pristine hemlock*
SOLITUDE: ☆ ☆ ☆ ☆	*forest, solitude, and interesting volcanic geology*

Although this hike is in Crater Lake National Park, I've seen more elk on it than people. You have two options for destinations: a rocky peak and a unique volcanic landscape. One is short on dramatic views, but both are long on forest, peace, and quiet. Note: *Pets are not allowed on this or any other trails in the park.*

It's amazing how easy it is to leave people behind in a national park. Hundreds of people drive by this trailhead every day without even noticing it, yet two interesting hikes start from it: this one and our OR 62 to Crater Lake Rim hike (page 47). Both introduce you to the part of the park that's away from the lake and, therefore, away from the RVs, gift shops, restaurants, lines, and so on. This one, especially, is all about solitude.

From the parking lot, head south on the Pacific Crest Trail, and in just a couple of minutes you'll encounter an interesting forest feature: a former quarry that supplied rocks for road-building and is now filled with young trees, all the same species and height, and all of them leaning about 15 degrees to the right—presumably because of wind and snow. Also in this area, look for a section of tree suspended about 20 feet off the ground between two other trees; when I scouted the trail, it was up there, and the rest of it was scattered all around the trail.

Forest attractions like this one will dominate your view for a while as you wind through the woods without much effort. Look for other features like logs that were cut to clear the trail (exposing their growth rings), decaying snags, the spiral pattern of wood in dead

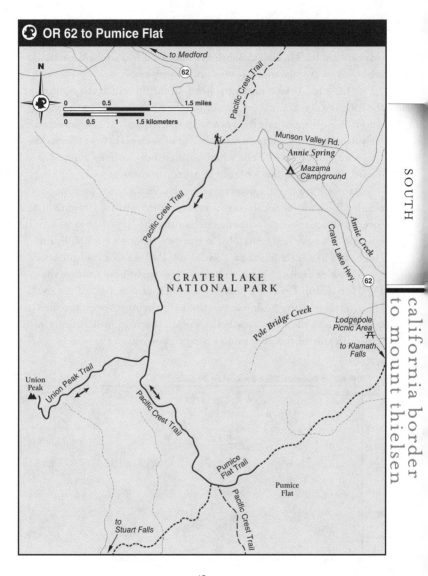

to Medford

62

N

| 0 | 0.5 | 1 | 1.5 miles |
| 0 | 0.5 | 1 | 1.5 kilometers |

Pacific Crest Trail

Munson Valley Rd.

Annie Spring

Mazama Campground

Pacific Crest Trail

Annie Creek

Crater Lake Hwy.

62

CRATER LAKE NATIONAL PARK

Pole Bridge Creek

Lodgepole Picnic Area

to Klamath Falls

Union Peak

Union Peak Trail

Pacific Crest Trail

Pumice Flat Trail

Pumice Flat

Pacific Crest Trail

to Stuart Falls

trees, and woodpecker holes in bark. Also look for blue diamonds up in the trees; they mark the trail for skiers and snowshoers, who love this easy grade. Those diamonds are about 20 feet up because the park gets an average of 44 feet of snow every year!

A little less than a mile out, head downhill, and at the bottom of the hill, see if you can spot an old roadbed heading off to the right. About five minutes past the roadbed, on the right, are two spectacularly decomposing snags—perfect cones of redwood. It was here that I once scared up several elk, who bounded away without making a sound. If you are quiet, you might get to see some as well.

Around the 2-mile mark, start back uphill a little, and then climb a little more steeply as you swing to the right (southwest) in a forest of huge mountain hemlocks—among the largest of these you'll ever see. The grade lessens a bit as you pass through a notch in the ridge, and at a little less than 3 miles you'll come to a trail junction.

If you're feeling up for a climb, stay straight here to leave the PCT for Union Peak, the best view in the southern part of the park. It's 2.6 miles to the peak. Climb gradually through forest for the first 0.8 mile, and then stay mostly flat for another 0.8 mile, traversing the south side of the peak and passing in and out of the woods. The

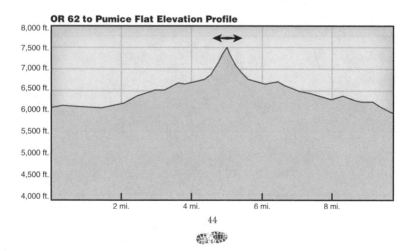

44

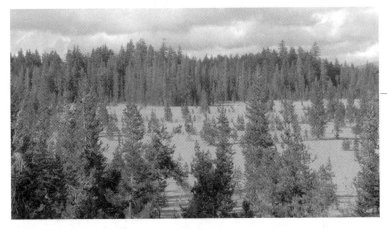

Pumice Flat, just off the PCT in Crater Lake National Park

trail then turns north, starts a series of switchbacks, and becomes quite steep and rocky; the last 0.6 mile gains a whopping 700 feet, and at times you'll find yourself using hands and feet to make progress. This route is shown on our elevation profile, bracketed by the Union Peak Trail junction.

If that doesn't sound like your bag, stay left and on the PCT at the junction, following a sign for Stuart Falls. The PCT climbs again after leaving the Union Peak Trail and then swings left (southeast) for a flat, forested stretch. Crater Peak, visible a few miles away to your left, is another hiking destination in the park.

In this meandering, mostly flat stretch of trail, look for a big gray snag with a tremendous burl eight feet off the ground, as well as a clump of eight or nine hemlocks bunched together on the left. There's also a view of craggy Union Peak to the right. Finally, 2.1 miles after the Union Peak junction, reach the Stuart Falls Trail heading south. This 50-foot plunge is worth a visit and has a campsite at its base, but at 2.5 miles from here, it makes for a long day.

Consider coming at it from other trailheads outside the park, or from the park's Lodgepole Picnic Area, which you'll reach if you continue on the Pumice Flat Trail. There's also great camping at Stuart Falls, so you might consider an overnight trip down there.

Stay on the PCT for just a few more minutes to reach a junction with the Pumice Flat Trail and its PCT register. It's fun to read these remarks, especially from the northbounders, who typically arrive in mid-August filled with dreams of showers, beer, and dinner at the Crater Lake Lodge. The Pumice Flat Trail, actually an abandoned road, drops for about a half mile onto the flats, which are filled with lodgepole pine and (according to park rangers) elk. These Pumice Flat are essentially valleys that were filled with volcanic spew when Mount Mazama erupted thousands of years ago.

The Pumice Flat Trail keeps going another 2.3 miles to a trailhead on OR 62 near the Lodgepole Picnic Area; you can do this hike as a one-way shuttle if you arrange for a second car there. Lodgepole is 3.5 miles south on OR 62 from the trailhead parking area described at the beginning of this hike.

DIRECTIONS From Medford, take OR 62 east for 75 miles to the PCT parking area on the right. Since this lot is 0.8 mile west of (thus outside) the park's south entrance station (Annie Spring Entrance Station), there's no fee or permit required to hike this trail, even though it is in the park.

PERMITS Since this trailhead is outside the park entrance station, parking is free.

GPS Trailhead Coordinates	5 OR 62 to Pumice Flat
UTM Zone (WGS84)	10T
Easting	566971
Northing	4746837
Latitude	N42° 52.272'
Longitude	W122° 10.804'

SCENERY: ✿ ✿ ✿	HIKING TIME: 2½ hours
TRAIL CONDITION: ✿ ✿ ✿	MAP: Crater Lake National Park
CHILDREN: ✿ ✿ ✿ ✿	OUTSTANDING FEATURES: *Quiet forest, a*
DIFFICULTY: ✿ ✿ ✿	*lovely creek, excellent campsites, and a sturdy climb*
SOLITUDE: ✿ ✿ ✿ ✿	*that makes a great view even better*
DISTANCE: 4.3 miles one-way	

How do you make the view of Crater Lake even better? The old-fashioned way: you earn it! Walk up there instead of driving, or use this seldom-visited section of the Pacific Crest Trail to explore the woods, enjoy some wildflowers, or add a secluded overnight backpack to your park visit. Note: No pets are allowed on this or any other trail in Crater Lake National Park.

🏃 From this section's founding in 1973, the PCT, incredibly, avoided the rim of Crater Lake, because horses are allowed on the trail but not up at the rim. To this day, if you hike the official PCT across Crater Lake National Park, you'll never lay your eyes on the lake.

But from the beginning, owing to simple common sense, hikers took off up the Dutton Creek Trail to the rim, then made their way along the Rim Drive and North Entrance Road, following them back to the PCT. Finally, in the 1990s, the Park Service relented and built a route along the rim called a "hiker's PCT," since horses are still not allowed up there. That rim hike is described in Hike 7 (page 52), and this one is a taste of the original trail.

You can do just the first half of this hike and not put in much effort at all, reaching a lovely creek in flower-filled meadows with lovely camping nearby—an excellent hike to take the kids on. Or you can do the whole thing and climb 1,000 feet in 2 miles to wind up at the rim. Or start at the top and walk down to the creek—suit yourself!

From the trailhead on OR 62, walk to and then across the highway, tending slightly to your right and looking for the trail reentering

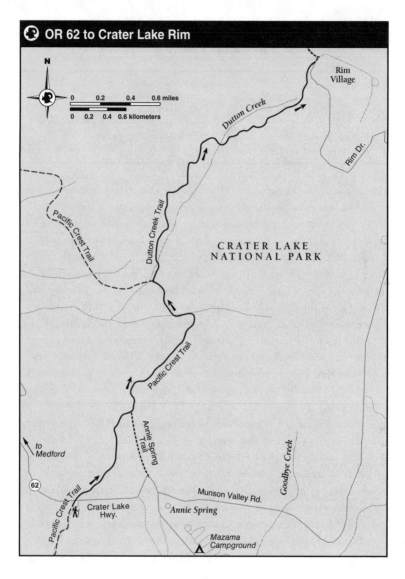

the woods on the north side of the road; you might spot a white or blue diamond on a tree or perhaps a rock cairn along the road. The trail starts out flat through trees and meadows; look for a big, impressive, hollowed-out snag on the right, at the head of a meadow about 0.2 mile in. Even if it's mid-August and northbound thru-hikers are on the move, you probably won't see them, since most take a "zero day" over at Mazama Village's campground, store, and restaurant. In part they do so because, after they leave there, they are looking at nearly 20 miles without a drop of water.

A total of 0.3 mile in, you start climbing a bit, and if you've just arrived from a lower elevation, you might feel short of breath. At 6,200 feet in elevation, it doesn't take much. You'll climb up the west side of a small ridge and, 0.6 mile from the road, intersect the Annie Spring Trail, which descends directly to Mazama Village.

After dropping again, you wind through a grassy hemlock forest with occasional views to the left of Watchman and Hillman Peaks, up on the rim. Yes, you're going down on your way up to the rim, and don't ask me why.

When you've gone 1.7 miles, you cross the first of three forks of Dutton Creek at the head of a grassy meadow, which, in early summer

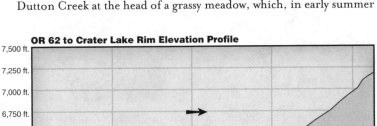

OR 62 to Crater Lake Rim Elevation Profile

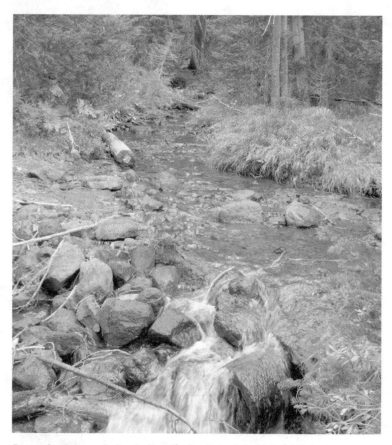

Dutton Creek crosses the Pacific Crest Trail in Crater Lake National Park; there is nice camping nearby.

(mid-July, around here) will be filled with flowers. At the second fork, 0.3 mile later, walk over a series of stones. And 0.1 mile after that, just before the westernmost fork, intersect the Dutton Creek Trail.

Beyond this, the PCT is just more of the same. A stake on the left marks a trail to lovely and often uncrowded campsites along the creek below the trail; *note that you need a free permit from the park to camp anywhere in the backcountry.*

Heading up the Dutton Creek Trail now, you can see that it's nothing too fancy: just a long series of switchbacks through the forest, crossing various forks of Dutton Creek several times, with little or nothing in the way of views—until the top, of course. It's 2.2 miles to Rim Drive. When you drop down briefly (again!) to a creek crossing, you've gone 1.3 miles and gained 400 feet, which means it's about to get steeper, as in climbing 650 feet over the last mile.

But you'll feel oh, so cool when you get to the rim, right? You can walk tall among the RV-driving picture takers, knowing that you had the strength to walk to the rim of Crater Lake!

DIRECTIONS From Medford, take OR 62 east for 75 miles to the PCT parking area on the right. Since this lot is 0.8 mile west of (thus outside) the park's south entrance station (Annie Spring Entrance Station), there's no fee or permit required to hike this trail, even though it is in the park.

PERMIT Since this trailhead is outside the park entrance station, parking is free.

GPS Trailhead Coordinates	6 OR 62 to Crater Lake Rim
UTM Zone (WGS84)	10T
Easting	566971
Northing	4746837
Latitude	N42° 52.272'
Longitude	W122° 10.804'

7 Crater Lake Rim

SCENERY: 🥾 🥾 🥾 🥾
TRAIL CONDITION: 🥾 🥾 🥾
CHILDREN: 🥾 🥾 🥾
DIFFICULTY: 🥾 🥾
SOLITUDE: 🥾
DISTANCE: 6.4 miles one-way

HIKING TIME: 3 hours
MAP: Crater Lake National Park
OUTSTANDING FEATURES: A 6-mile-wide, 1,900-foot-deep lake, 1,000 feet below you, with mountains all around. Need anything else?

This bit of trail is so amazing that it has become part of the PCT. So many people were walking off the original trail to see Oregon's most stupendous site that the Park Service built this section of trail as a "hiker's PCT." And you'll see why, as you meander along the rim of the caldera, enjoying view after view after view. Note: *Pets are not allowed in the backcountry (on trail or off) of Crater Lake National Park, and they must be leashed elsewhere in the park.*

As the PCT winds its way across Oregon, it passes in and out of amazing scenery—none more amazing than Crater Lake. It also passes through solitary areas and crowded ones—none more crowded than Crater Lake. Still, this easy walk is the best way to experience the Crater Lake Rim, because 99 percent of the throngs will stick to the road and parking areas, while you're hiking from one private viewing area to the next.

Before the 1990s, when the PCT still stayed 1,000 feet below the rim, hikers would walk up the Dutton Creek Trail to the Rim Village, then make their way along the road or off-trail to the North Entrance Road. But during the 1990s, the Park Service built the trail you're about to walk, a one-way 6-miler that parallels the road. (Equestrians must stick to the official PCT.) On this trail, you can do as little as you want, or use a second car to set up a shuttle, or do a 12-mile round-trip that should take no more than five hours. (The hike up the Dutton Creek Trail is described in Hike 6, page 47.)

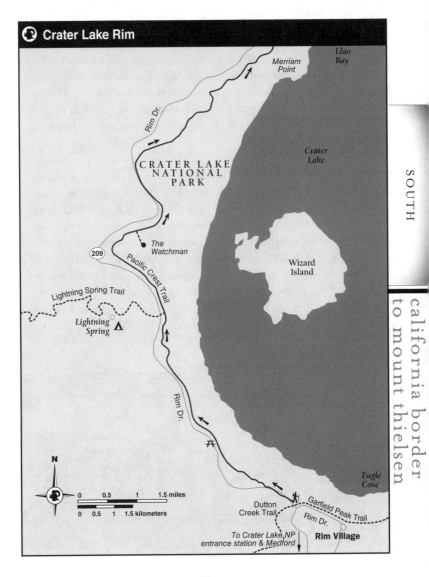

Llao Bay

Merriam Point

CRATER LAKE NATIONAL PARK

Crater Lake

Rim Dr.

209

Pacific Crest Trail

The Watchman

Lightning Spring Trail

Lightning Spring

Wizard Island

Rim Dr.

N

0   0.5   1   1.5 miles

0   0.5   1   1.5 kilometers

Eagle Cove

Dutton Creek Trail

Garfield Peak Trail

Rim Dr.

To Crater Lake NP entrance station & Medford

Rim Village

SOUTH

california border to mount thielsen

Starting at the Rim Village, just walk up to the rim and turn left, along a stone wall with the lake on your right. Try to wrap your head around the distances involved: it's 6 miles to the other side of the lake, and the distance from you to the lake (about 1,000 feet in most places) is about half that from the surface to the bottom! And by the way, it's a caldera, not a crater. Mount Mazama imploded to form it—the deepest lake in the United States and one of the 10 deepest in the world.

When you get to the top of the access road, the trail drops down 0.1 mile to the first of many cliffs; needless to say, be very careful here. At 0.2 mile, you reach the first of several parking areas along the road, and the trail starts back up with views of Wizard Island, a cinder cone that built up after the caldera was formed; you can take a highly recommended boat ride to it during the summer.

The next mile takes you away from the road, up a hill of a hundred feet or so, to several spots where you're even more exposed to the edge of the cliffs; this is not a hike for folks afraid of heights! At 1.1 miles, you'll be back at the road with a big parking area. Looking south from this area, you can see Mount McLoughlin and prominent

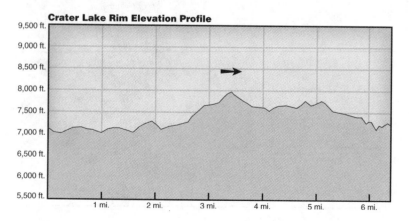

Crater Lake Rim Elevation Profile

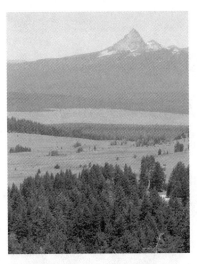

The view north from the Crater Lake Rim includes Mount Thielsen, the next destination north on the PCT.

Devils Peak, a PCT landmark described in Hike 4 (page 36); to the PCT hiker, that's about 22 miles away.

Check out some of the interpretive signs in this parking area, and then head up some switchbacks and over another hill, this one reaching as high as 7,319 feet above sea level (about 200 feet above the last parking area). Looking ahead here, see The Watchman with its lookout tower; you can go there in a bit if you'd like.

At 2.2 miles, drop down a steep little pitch to the road again and have your closest view of Wizard Island. Find the trail at the far end of the parking lot, where it heads up the hill right before a sign saying "Lightning Spring 500 feet." Reach the Lightning Spring Picnic Area in 0.2 mile, and across the road is the trailhead of the same name for another access trail from the official PCT down the hill. It leads to a spring and campground in 0.8 mile, but you need a permit from the park to camp there.

From the Lightning Spring Picnic Area, your current route bends out to the west to get around The Watchman. It also climbs steadily, gaining 500 feet in 0.7 mile to a junction with the trail to the peak's summit. Since you're up here, go on up to the summit, which is 0.4 mile and 300 feet above you; it's a well-graded climb to the peak at 8,013 feet. The views stretch from California's Mount Shasta north to the Three Sisters, sticking up to the left of

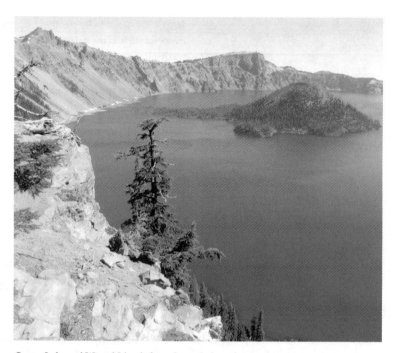

Crater Lake and Wizard Island, from the trail along the rim

needle-pointed Mount Thielsen—and there's the lake, of course.
The Watchman got its name from an event in 1886, when a group of
engineers was placed here to take observations while another group
toured the lake by boat, taking soundings of its depth.

Back on the trail below The Watchman, traverse a boulder field
before dropping down to a big parking area with more vault toilets and
interpretive signs. At this point, if you've gone up to The Watchman,
you've hiked a total of 4.1 miles since leaving Rim Village. Pick up the
trail at the far end of the lot's fences, just past the toilet, and enjoy
1.2 miles of open strolling around the west side of Hillman Peak, the

highest spot on the rim, named for one of the lake's "discoverers" in 1853. Along this stretch, you start to get views north to Diamond Lake, Mount Thielsen, and the Three Sisters, as well as the immense Pumice Flat that northbound PCT hikers have to look forward to.

At 5.9 miles, the trail empties out onto the road around the corner from another parking area. Go 100 yards and look for where the trail resumes on a dirt mound at the far end of the lot; walk up that and aim for a clump of gnarled trees. At the next parking area, in 0.1 mile, pick up the trail at the end of a stone guardrail, just before another clump of trees.

Finally, after one last little hump, reach a parking area with road signs for the Rim Drive continuing east. At this point, you're done. The PCT crosses Rim Drive just east of the North Entrance Road and then heads north from a rock cairn for 11.5 miles of viewless, waterless, pumice-filled joy to OR 138. Thru-hikers who started at the Rim Village have to walk the 6 miles you just hiked, those 11.5 miles, and then another 8 miles to Thielsen Creek before they cross a drop of water. Aren't you glad you aren't doing that with a full pack?

DIRECTIONS From Medford, travel east on OR 62 for 76 miles to the south entrance (Annie Spring Entrance Station) to Crater Lake National Park. The entrance fee is $10 per vehicle and is good for 10 days. Follow Munson Valley Road and then Rim Drive 7.5 miles to Rim Village, where parking is abundant.

PERMIT The park charges a $10 entrance fee.

GPS Trailhead Coordinates	7 Crater Lake Rim
UTM Zone (WGS84)	10T
Easting	569562
Northing	4751404
Latitude	N42° 54.725'
Longitude	W122° 8.867'

8 Mount Thielsen Loop

SCENERY: ✿ ✿ ✿ ✿	HIKING TIME: *3 days*
TRAIL CONDITION: ✿ ✿ ✿	MAP: *USFS PCT Oregon: Southern Section or*
CHILDREN: ✿	*USFS Mount Thielsen Wilderness*
DIFFICULTY: ✿ ✿ ✿ ✿	OUTSTANDING FEATURES: *Staggering views*
SOLITUDE: ✿ ✿ ✿	*from a peak above 9,000 feet, high-elevation forest,*
DISTANCE: *21.6 miles*	*and camping by a tumbling mountain stream*

Even if you aren't into mountain climbing and don't want to tackle "The Lightning Rod of the Cascades," this hike is worth the effort for big views and a chance to camp way up in the hills. Only about a third of these miles are on the Pacific Crest Trail, but they are not your average miles. There are a lot of trails in this small area, and the hike suggested here is my favorite introduction to it.

🚶🚶 This hike starts out with one of the most fantastically confusing trail signs you're likely to see. It's one thing when signs have the wrong distances or something, but this one seems designed to make you stop and scratch your head. You've got Trail 1448, a "connection" to Trail 1448, and then, 4 miles ahead, *another* Trail 1448.

The reality is that there's a small loop from here that leads to the same place, so turn left and follow Trail 1448, the Howlock Mountain Trail. It passes under the highway at 0.2 mile, then a mile later reaches Trail 1458, the Spruce Ridge Trail. Ignore that and keep on trucking, though dry, dusty woods on a trail made wide by horse traffic. A welcome patch of green comes into view when Timothy Meadows opens up on the far side of Thielsen Creek, about 3 miles up. Ignore a side trail to the left, and a few minutes later cross the creek in a lovely grassy area, most welcome after the viewless dust bowl you've been coming through. There's no bridge here (though a small log spans the creek), but even if you have to wade it's no problem.

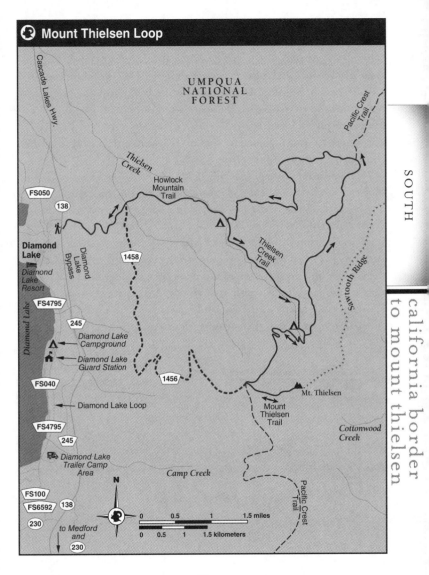

Mount Thielsen Loop

UMPQUA
NATIONAL
FOREST

Cascade Lakes Hwy.

Thielsen Creek

Pacific Crest Trail

Howlock Mountain Trail

FS050

138

Diamond Lake

Diamond Lake Resort

Diamond Lake Bypass

1458

Thielsen Creek Trail

Sawtooth Ridge

FS4795

Diamond Lake

245

Diamond Lake Campground

Diamond Lake Guard Station

1456

FS040

Diamond Lake Loop

Mt. Thielsen

Mount Thielsen Trail

Cottonwood Creek

FS4795

245

Diamond Lake Trailer Camp Area

Camp Creek

N

Pacific Crest Trail

FS100

FS6592

138

230

to Medford and

230

0   0.5   1   1.5 miles

0   0.5   1   1.5 kilometers

About 30 yards past the creek you see the Thielsen Creek Trail (#1449) heading up to the right; take that, and start to climb with a little more purpose; the next 2.2 miles gains about 900 feet, but the views of Mount Thielsen finally start about halfway up, when you hit a flat stretch of pumice. As you arrive at the PCT, look for campsites below you and to the right. There are also campsites above the trail to the left just before the creek crossing. My advice is to make this area home for two nights. The view of Thielsen and the sound of the creek make for a sublime setting.

The next morning, especially if you want to go up Thielsen, start early to beat the heat and crowds. And even if you aren't a climber, follow the first part of this route for some great scenery. Turn right (south) on the PCT, hop across the creek, and follow the trail's slow climb through a thick forest that usually has snow in it well into July. You finally pop out into the open and, 1.2 miles past the creek, round a ridge where the views are amazing. Next is a flat mile of about the most scenic trail you can hike, with the west face of Thielsen right above you, Diamond Lake down below, and a flower-filled alpine wonderland all around—fantastic stuff.

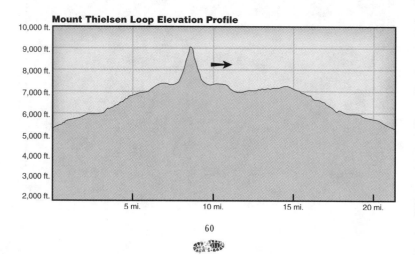

60

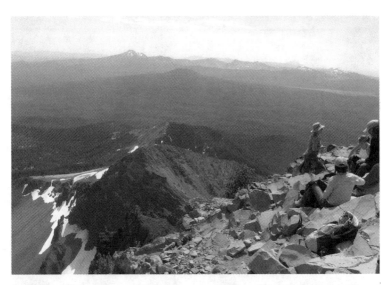

Relaxing on Chicken Point, just below the summit of Mount Thielsen with a view of the peaks around Crater Lake

When you get to the Mt. Thielsen Trail (#1456), you need to make a decision. Climbing Mount Thielsen, though popular and nontechnical, is a challenging and potentially hazardous endeavor. It's quite steep, rocky, dry, and remote. Even if you don't go all the way to the summit, you'll be on or near very high clifftops, and you'll need to climb on both loose and solid rock. Don't go alone, take plenty of water, and bring a cell phone for emergencies.

Now, if I haven't scared you off, head on up. There's a pretty clear trail, especially at first, and even if it splits, all the options go to the same place. Basically, "up" is the right way. Eventually you have to choose between more solid rock to the left and scree to the right; stay left and look for a little chute up ahead, on the south side of the peak. At the top of that chute is a big, wide ledge that some

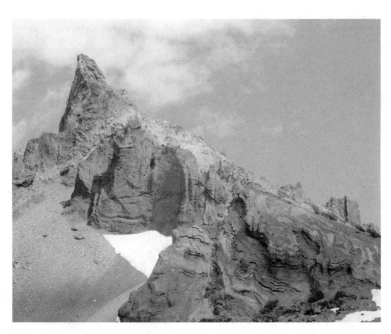

Mount Thielsen, the "Lightning Rod of the Cascades": The climbing route is basically the right skyline.

people call "Chicken Point," because it's the end of the climb for a lot of people. Count me among the chickens, as I did not tackle the last 80 feet of real rock climbing to the tiny summit. Anyway, even a chicken's view is outstanding; you can see the surface of Crater Lake, as well as the island known as Phantom Ship. Also look for Mounts Shasta and McLoughlin to the south, and if you go to the far end of the ledge you can see north to red Tipsoo Peak in the foreground (see Hike 9, page 64) and Mount Jefferson off in the distance. Note that from Shasta to Jefferson is about 225 miles! See if you can find your tent down there in the trees as well.

Head back down the way you came up (or whatever way you can do it safely), and when you get to the PCT, backtrack to camp. You might spend another night there, perhaps splashing in the creek. Then, the next morning, either go down the way you came up (5.6 miles) or put in some more time on the PCT and make a 10-mile return. Do the latter particularly if you want to combine this hike with the Tipsoo Peak and Maidu Lake hike (Hike 9, page 64). That would be a great three-nighter!

From the creek, it's 3 mostly flat miles north on the PCT to a pumice flat with great views of Thielsen, Sawtooth Ridge, and Tipsoo Peak. The trail wraps around the flat to its junction with the Howlock Mountain Trail (#1448), where you started this hike. Head down that for 7.2 miles to the trailhead. Or if you're connecting to Tipsoo and Maidu, you've already knocked those 7.2 miles off that trek, and you're now 1.7 miles from the Tipsoo turnoff and 6.8 miles from the Maidu Lake Trail.

DIRECTIONS The Howlock Mountain Trailhead lies just off OR 138, 4.2 miles north of its intersection with OR 230. That intersection is 79 miles east of Roseburg on 138 and 82 miles east of Medford on 230. Traveling north on 138, look for a sign that says "Diamond Lake Recreation Area and FS 4795." The trailhead is 0.3 mile down that road on the left; it shares a parking lot with the Diamond Lake Corrals. A Northwest Forest Pass is required.

PERMITS A Northwest Forest Pass is required.

GPS Trailhead Coordinates	8 Mount Thielsen Loop
UTM Zone (WGS84)	10T
Easting	570422
Northing	4781577
Latitude	N43° 11.021'
Longitude	W122° 8.006'

9 Tipsoo Peak and Maidu Lake

SCENERY: ✿ ✿ ✿ ✿	HIKING TIME: *3 days*
TRAIL CONDITION: ✿ ✿ ✿	MAP: *USFS* PCT Oregon: Southern Section *or*
CHILDREN: ✿	USFS Mount Thielsen Wilderness
DIFFICULTY: ✿ ✿ ✿ ✿	OUTSTANDING FEATURES: *Mountain streams,*
SOLITUDE: ✿ ✿ ✿ ✿	*panoramic views, and camping by a beautiful lake*
DISTANCE: *30.4 miles*	

Don't be scared off by the length of this hike. Think of it as three possible routes in one: either a moderate climb to camping at Thielsen Creek (about 7 miles round-trip), a strenuous trek to Tipsoo Peak's amazing views (17 miles) or a long two- or three-day excursion to Maidu Lake. You can also combine it with the Mount Thielsen Loop for a real multiday adventure. And for what it's worth, this hike visits the highest point on the PCT in Oregon and Washington.

🏃 This hike will take you from one of the more populated areas around, Diamond Lake, to one of the loneliest, highest, and driest stretches of Oregon's Pacific Crest Trail. In fact, the suggested hike here is so long partly because once you get to the PCT, there's neither water nor camping for several miles either way. But the views and the solitude more than make up for the length and hassle.

Things are somewhat confusing at the trailhead because there seem to be multiple trails going the same way, and in fact there are. What you're after is Trail 1448, the Howlock Mountain Trail, which after 0.2 mile passes under OR 138. Stay with Trail 1448 for another mile to an intersection with Trail 1458, the Spruce Ridge Trail. Stay straight on Trail 1448, and after 2 more miles, cross Thielsen Creek on the edge of beautiful Timothy Meadows. Walk along the creek for almost a mile before crossing it. You could camp under some trees in this area, if you don't want to haul your pack the rest of the

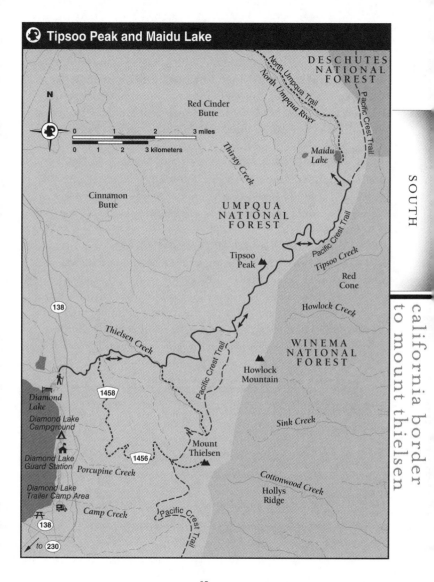

DESCHUTES
NATIONAL
FOREST

North Umpqua Trail

North Umpqua River

Pacific Crest Trail

Red Cinder
Butte

N

0   1   2   3 miles

0   1   2   3 kilometers

Maidu
Lake

Thirsty Creek

SOUTH

Cinnamon
Butte

UMPQUA
NATIONAL
FOREST

Pacific Crest Trail

Tipsoo
Peak

Tipsoo Creek

Red
Cone

Howlock Creek

138

Thielsen Creek

Pacific Crest Trail

WINEMA
NATIONAL
FOREST

Howlock
Mountain

california border
to mount thielsen

1458

Diamond
Lake

Diamond Lake
Campground

Sink Creek

Diamond Lake
Guard Station

1456

Mount
Thielsen

Porcupine Creek

Cottonwood Creek

Diamond Lake
Trailer Camp Area

Hollys
Ridge

Camp Creek

Pacific Crest Trail

138

to 230

way up the hill. Just make sure you camp at least 100 feet from trails and water. This also makes for a nice picnic and turnaround spot; a round-trip hike to here is 6.8 miles with a total gain of just 800 feet.

Beyond the creek, the climb resumes for 3.6 more miles (and 1,200 feet) to the PCT. About 2 miles up, you round a ridge and trek back to the east, at which point 8,324-foot Howlock Mountain (named for a local Paiute chief) will dominate the view ahead.

Intersect the PCT on the edge of a pumice flat with a big-time view, from Mount Thielsen on your right to Sawtooth Ridge and Howlock Mountain in front of you. Snow lingers up here into July most years; if you're here in early summer and seasonal creeks are flowing, you could camp here. The whole area goes dry as soon as the snow is gone though.

Turn left (north) onto the PCT, and climb for 0.4 mile to a saddle. Then traverse north through meadows and pumice where posts occasionally mark the trail. When the saddle is 1.3 miles behind you, cross over another, inconspicuous saddle that is significant for your journey in two ways. One, it's the turnoff point to climb reddish Tipsoo Peak (8,034 feet) to your left, and two, at 7,560 feet, it is the highest point on the PCT in Oregon and Washington.

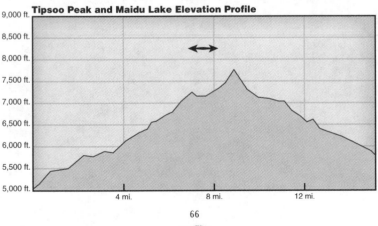

Tipsoo Peak and Maidu Lake Elevation Profile

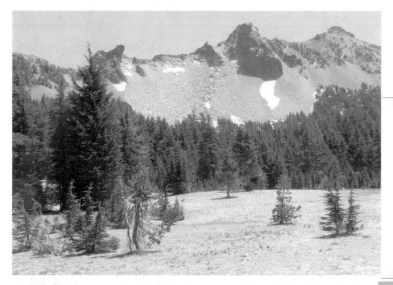

Howlock Mountain and a pumice flat from the highest stretch of the PCT in the Pacific Northwest

There's no trail to Tipsoo, but it's sitting right there. The peak on the left is the higher of the two, and the peak's right side offers the most gradual climb. It's rocky going, but the view is worth the half-hour slog. Mount Thielsen dominates to the south with Diamond Lake visible to the right of it. To the north, it's possible to just make out (from right to left) Mount Bachelor as well as South and Middle Sister. For the northbound PCT hiker, South Sister is about 100 miles ahead. There are whitebark pine (now on the endangered species list) all around the top of Tipsoo Peak.

Back down on the trail at the saddle, you can turn back (you're 8.8 miles from the trailhead and 5.4 miles from Thielsen Creek) or put in another 6 downhill miles to Maidu Lake. Along the way, you'll get views of the colorful north side of Tipsoo Peak (*tipsoo*, by the way, is Chinook for "hair") and east to Miller Lake and Red Cone. Otherwise, it's an easy descent with little to see.

Five miles down from the saddle, reach the Maidu Lake Trail, and take it left for 0.9 mile to the lake. There's plenty of camping on the near shore, but if you happen to get there in July or early August there will also be a maddening swarm of mosquitoes. Some old maps show a shelter at this location, but it's long gone.

Maidu Lake is the headwaters of the North Umpqua River, one of the more beautiful rivers in Oregon, as well as a sought-after steelhead fishing destination. I mention this because the North Umpqua Trail starts at the lake and follows the river for 79 miles, passing campgrounds, lakes, and hot springs along the way—something to think about when you're done with your PCT adventures.

DIRECTIONS The Howlock Mountain Trailhead lies just off OR 138, 4.2 miles north of its intersection with OR 230. That intersection is 79 miles east of Roseburg on 138 and 82 miles east of Medford on 230. Traveling north on 138, look for a sign that says "Diamond Lake Recreation Area and FS 4795." The trailhead is 0.3 mile down that road on the left; it shares a parking lot with the Diamond Lake Corrals. A Northwest Forest Pass is required.

PERMITS A Northwest Forest Pass is required.

GPS Trailhead Coordinates	9 Tipsoo Peak and Maidu Lake
UTM Zone (WGS84)	10T
Easting	570422
Northing	4781577
Latitude	N43° 11.021'
Longitude	W122° 8.006'

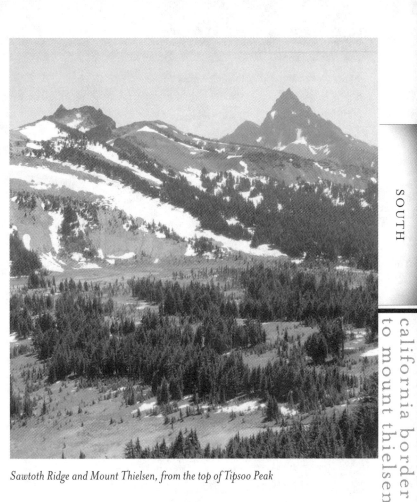

Sawtoth Ridge and Mount Thielsen, from the top of Tipsoo Peak

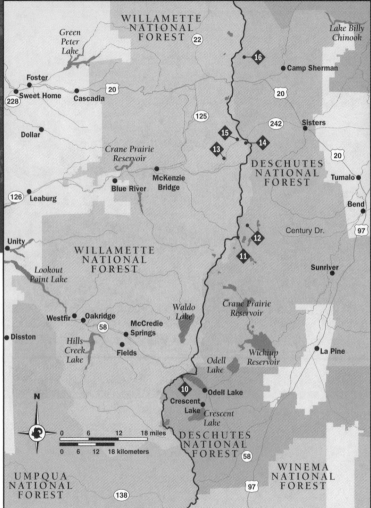

WILLAMETTE
NATIONAL
FOREST
22

Green
Peter
Lake

16

Camp Sherman

Foster

20

Sweet Home   Cascadia
228

20

125

242   Sisters

Dollar

15

13   14

20

Crane Prairie
Reservoir

DESCHUTES
NATIONAL
FOREST

McKenzie
Bridge

Tumalo

Blue River

126   Leaburg

Bend

97

Unity

WILLAMETTE
NATIONAL
FOREST

12

Century Dr.

11

Lookout
Point Lake

Sunriver

Westfir   Oakridge
58

Waldo
Lake

Crane Prairie
Reservoir

Disston

McCredie
Springs

Hills
Creek
Lake

Fields

Wickiup
Reservoir

La Pine

Odell
Lake

N

10

Odell Lake

Crescent
Lake   Crescent
Lake

0   6   12   18 miles

0   6   12   18 kilometers

DESCHUTES
NATIONAL
FOREST
58

UMPQUA
NATIONAL
FOREST

WINEMA
NATIONAL
FOREST

138

97

2

CENTRAL

Willamette Pass to Santiam Pass

10 Rosary Lakes to Maiden Peak Shelter (*page 72*)

11 Mink Lake Basin (*page 76*)

12 Wickiup Plain to Sisters Mirror Lake (*page 81*)

13 Obsidian Loop (*page 86*)

14 Lava Camp Lake to Collier Glacier View (*page 92*)

15 Little Belknap Crater (*page 98*)

16 Three-Fingered Jack (*page 102*)

10 Rosary Lakes
to Maiden Peak Shelter

SCENERY: ☆ ☆
TRAIL CONDITION: ☆ ☆ ☆ ☆
CHILDREN: ☆ ☆ ☆ ☆
DIFFICULTY: ☆ ☆
SOLITUDE: ☆ ☆ ☆
DISTANCE: 6.6 miles to North Rosary Lake (out-and-back), 11.6 miles to shelter (out-and-back)

HIKING TIME: 3½ hours
MAP: *USFS* Middle Fork Ranger District
OUTSTANDING FEATURES: *A quiet walk through shady forest to three mountain lakes, with a nice view and hidden cabin if you want to go farther*

This is an easy-to-reach, easy-to-hike leg stretcher that's perfect for an afternoon outing or a simple overnighter with the family. And if you put in a few more miles, you can spend the night in a wonderful cabin.

The hike up to the Rosary Lakes is one of the more popular in the area, and it's no wonder. Pacific Crest Trail hikers tend to blow on through, however, since most of them just stopped at Odell Lake to rest and resupply. Chances are, you'll see other folks on the trail, and you won't care.

The first 2 miles or so are about as gradual and mellow as a hike can be. There's not much to see, other than big trees and the occasional glimpse of Odell Lake off to the right. The total trip to Lower Rosary Lake is 2.4 miles and gains a little more than 500 feet.

For reference along the way, at 0.9 mile, the trail turns to the north in a flat section and enters a younger forest with much less ground cover. At 1.4 miles, it reenters the more diverse forest, and at 1.6 miles look for a gigantic hemlock snag covered with woodpecker holes. Finally, just past 1.8 miles, round the eastern edge of a minor ridge, and turn north, leaving the sounds of cars and trains behind.

When you get to the first lake at 2.4 miles, look for good swimming off a rockslide to your left and campsites on an around-the-lake

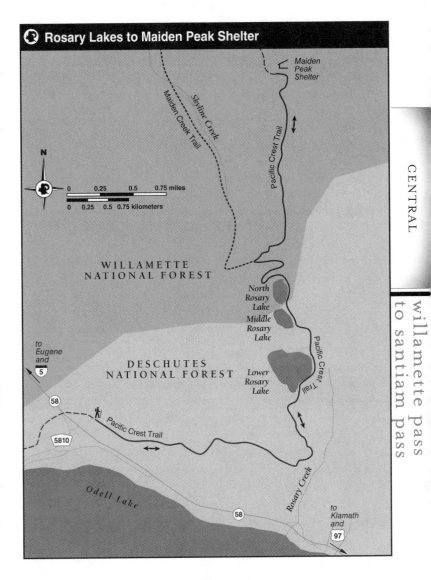

N

0   0.25   0.5   0.75 miles

0   0.25   0.5 0.75 kilometers

Maiden
Peak
Shelter

Maiden Creek Trail

Skyline Creek

Pacific Crest Trail

WILLAMETTE
NATIONAL FOREST

North
Rosary
Lake

Middle
Rosary
Lake

Pacific Crest Trail

to
Eugene
and
5

DESCHUTES
NATIONAL FOREST

Lower
Rosary
Lake

58

Pacific Crest Trail

5810

Odell Lake

58

Rosary Creek

to
Klamath
and
97

path. Other good campsites are along the right side of the lake, across the PCT from the shore.

Past this first lake, climb gently again, back in the forest, and 0.3 mile past the lower lake, arrive at Middle Rosary Lake, which is the most scenic of all. It's surprisingly deep, for the elevation, and Pulpit Rock across the way makes a handsome backdrop. There's a fine campsite between Middle and North Rosary Lakes, a distance of only 100 yards.

Now, if you want to get a nicer view of the lakes and possibly spend the night in some unique accommodations, put in some more mileage north on the PCT. And don't ask me why the lakes are named Lower, Middle, and North; it seems like that last one ought to be Upper.

Continue north beyond North Rosary Lake, climbing 300 feet in a mile to Maiden Peak Saddle, with lake-filled views to the south. After a smidge more climbing, continue north along the east side of a ridge for a total of 1.6 miles.

Just before the PCT crosses to the west side of the ridge, look for a cairn on the trail at the edge of an open flat. Across that flat is the Maiden Peak Shelter, built in 1999 by the Eugene Chapter of the

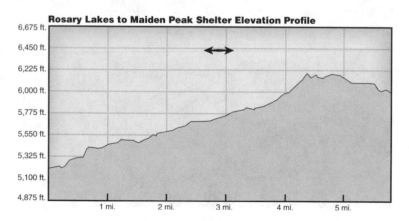

Rosary Lakes to Maiden Peak Shelter Elevation Profile

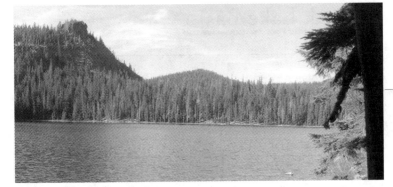

Lower Rosary Lake from the PCT

Oregon Nordic Club. Inside (it isn't locked) you'll find a woodstove and sleeping space for a dozen or more people. It's quite comfy and will spare you having to haul a tent—if you get there in time for a spot!

DIRECTIONS From I-5 just south of Eugene, follow OR 58 for 62 miles east to the Willamette Pass Ski Area. Go another 0.2 mile east, then turn left, following a sign for PCT Trailhead. After 100 feet, turn right on a gravel road, and follow it 0.1 mile to the end of the road. There's an outhouse here, and no fee is required.

PERMIT None required.

GPS Trailhead Coordinates	10 Rosary Lakes to Maiden Peak Shelter
UTM zone (WGS84)	10T
Easting	578410
Northing	4827494
Latitude	N43° 35.777'
Longitude	W122° 1.714'

SCENERY: 🐾 🐾	HIKING TIME: *15 hours (at least one night recommended)*
TRAIL CONDITION: 🐾 🐾 🐾 🐾	
CHILDREN: 🐾 🐾	MAP: *Green Trails* Three Sisters
DIFFICULTY: 🐾	OUTSTANDING FEATURES: *Seemingly endless forest and countless lakes with very few people around*
SOLITUDE: 🐾 🐾 🐾 🐾	
DISTANCE: *24 miles out-and-back to Mink Lake, plus up to several miles exploring the lake basin*	

Everybody knows about the Three Sisters Wilderness—or they think they do. What they know about is the northern half, the one with the big peaks. But the southern half is a giant, forested, lake-filled batch of solitude. The highlight is the area around Mink Lake, roughly 200 acres and 12 miles from the nearest road. Use this easy hike to reach a camp in the area, to explore all around—and leave the crowds up north.

🚶🚶 Okay, before you do this hike, get out a map and look at the southern half of Three Sisters Wilderness. Look at all the lakes! It's amazing. I met a thru-hiker on the PCT in here one time, and when I asked which lake we were nearby, he first said that I was the only person he'd seen for days, and then added, "Man, I've seen so many lakes the last two days, I don't know or care which is which!" That about sums it up.

Another thing to know before you go: this hike is easy! Sure, it's 12 miles to Mink Lake, but with a total elevation gain of a little more than 1,000 feet—a third of that in the first mile.

So, from the Elk Lake Trailhead, take Trail 3 to the left, and in just a few minutes enter a large area that burned about a decade ago. As you can see, it was a pretty catastrophic fire, but it opened up the area for views: You can spot South Sister (and the climbers' trail headed for the summit) as well as Broken Top and Mount Bachelor. After a mile of climbing through this, hit the PCT, where you go left,

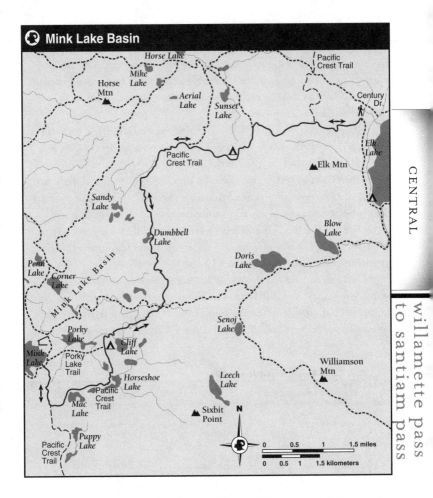

Horse Lake

Mike Lake

Horse Mtn

Aerial Lake

Sunset Lake

Pacific Crest Trail

Century Dr.

Elk Lake

Pacific Crest Trail

Elk Mtn

Sandy Lake

Dumbbell Lake

Blow Lake

Doris Lake

Penn Lake

Corner Lake

Mink Lake Basin

Porky Lake

Cliff Lake

Senoj Lake

Williamson Mtn

Mink Lake

Porky Lake Trail

Horseshoe Lake

Pacific Crest Trail

Leech Lake

Mac Lake

N

Puppy Lake

Sixbit Point

Pacific Crest Trail

0   0.5   1   1.5 miles
0   0.5   1   1.5 kilometers

and in moments reenter the forest. What a difference, eh? Get used to this forest cover; you are in it the rest of the way.

The trail flattens out now, passes a trail on the right and a meadow on the left a mile later, and then starts to climb slightly before, at 3.2 miles total, there's a sad little trail-side campsite next to a tiny creek. This is the kind of site a thru-hiker would drop into right at dark after a 35-mile day, but we can do better. The site does mark your entrance into the Island Meadow area, so named because in the middle of the big meadow is an island of trees, and in the middle of that a tiny pond.

Keep truckin' on the PCT, climbing ever so slightly for the next mile and a half, the main highlight being a comical sign situation at a trail junction. The sign on the left says it's #4337, the one on the right says it's #3515, and the map says it's #3517—and there's no #4337 anywhere to be found. Stick with the PCT, and a half mile past that junction, start a gradual, 3-mile descent to the junction with Trail #14 on the left. (If you have a second car, this is a good way out for a shuttle.) Halfway down, at 6 miles from the trailhead, there's great camping at scenic Dumbbell Lake.

If you're not up for the whole 12-mile trek to Mink Lake, 9 miles will get you to Cliff Lake, which is a beautiful spot with excellent tent sites, a shelter, and terrific swimming. There's no sign for it, but when you see, at 9 miles, the Porky Lake Trail on your right, look

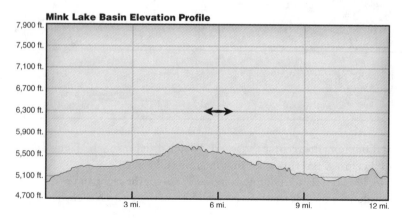

Mink Lake Basin Elevation Profile

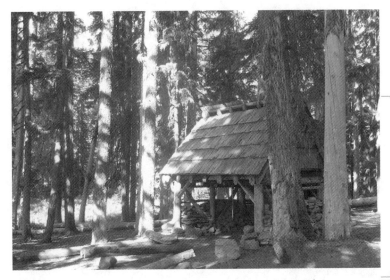

The shelter at Deep Lake, where there's excellent camping just off the PCT, dates to at least 1955.

over your left shoulder for a trail going along a rockslide; you can just make out Cliff Lake through there, about 100 yards away. See if you can find the 1955 graffiti in the shelter.

Beyond that junction on the PCT, it's all lakes, all the time. First up is Horseshoe Lake on the left, with a sweet campsite, then Merrill Lake, large Mac Lake, and S Lake. At S Lake, which is 2.3 miles past Cliff Lake, take the Mink Lake Trail on the right, and after going over a small rise (where you can catch another glimpse of South Sister), drop down to giant Mink Lake in less than a mile.

There is a trail all the way around Mink Lake, and if you go right on, you'll find a sprawling campsite with another historic shelter in a quarter mile. In fact, you can find all 10 named lakes within a couple miles of Mink Lake, most of them connected by trails, some of which may not be maintained, making them adventurous. But you like adventure, right? My advice is to camp in the area with a good map, compass, and GPS receiver, plus a fishing rod, and head out exploring. Oh, and legend has it that there are monsters living in Mud Lake.

To head back, take the trail past Porky Lake and back up to the PCT at the Cliff Lake junction. From there, you're 9 miles from the car at Elk Lake Trailhead, where milkshakes wait across the road in the Elk Lake Resort's cafe. You deserve it; you're an explorer of little-known wilderness lakes!

DIRECTIONS From Bend, follow Century Drive (aka Cascade Lakes Highway), which is signed for Mount Bachelor, for 30 miles to the trailhead on the right; it's across the road from the entrance to Elk Lake Resort.

PERMIT A Northwest Forest Pass is required.

GPS Trailhead Coordinates	11 Mink Lake Basin
UTM Zone (WGS84)	10T
Easting	595276
Northing	4870675
Latitude	N43° 58.982'
Longitude	W121° 48.719'

12 Wickiup Plain to Sisters Mirror Lake

SCENERY: ✿ ✿ ✿ ✿	HIKING TIME: *9 hours*
TRAIL CONDITION: ✿ ✿ ✿	MAP: *Green Trails Three Sisters or*
CHILDREN: ✿ ✿ ✿ ✿	*USFS Three Sisters Wilderness*
DIFFICULTY: ✿ ✿	OUTSTANDING FEATURES: *Sparkling moun-*
SOLITUDE: ✿ ✿	*tain lakes, moonscape plains, towering peaks, and*
DISTANCE: *15.1 miles*	*volcanic craters*

This loop through the South Sister area is dramatic in several ways. It's volcanic, alpine, forested, moonlike, and watery at the same time. It can be a long day hike or a simple overnight or serve as the basis of a multiday exploration of the Three Sisters Wilderness. All this, and the total elevation gain is barely 100 feet per mile!

🚶 Shortly after leaving the trailhead, enter the Three Sisters Wilderness and enjoy a little warm-up stretch of nearly flat forest. At 0.5 mile, stay straight ahead at a junction with the Elk-Devils Trail, which we will return on. Hop over Sink Creek here, and then round the southern edge of Kokostick Butte (*kokostick* is Chinook for "wood-pecker") and, at 1.3 miles, pass a pond to the right. All this is on a trail that hardly seems to climb at all.

Just past 2.5 miles, traverse a clearing with a view left to Koosah Mountain (*koosah* is Chinook for "sky"), and at 3.5 miles reach the Pacific Crest Trail. The trail you've come in on continues ahead as the Nash Lake Trail, but turn left here onto the PCT, headed for Sisters Mirror Lake. Before you get there, I suggest you take a trail heading off to the right; Sisters Mirror is only one of several lakes in this area, and frankly it's not even the nicest. This little trail, which isn't on the map, goes over a small rise to the first of these other lakes; it seems to have no name, but it does have a nice campsite.

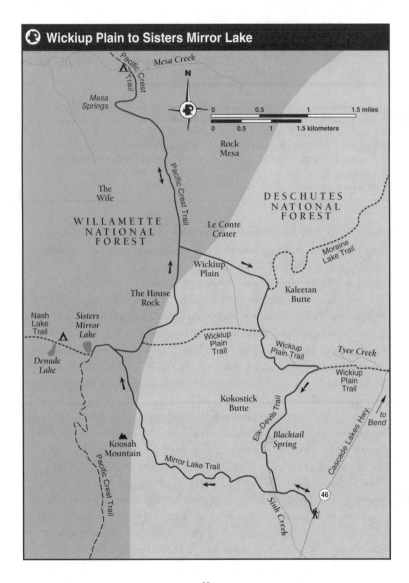

Wickiup Plain to Sisters Mirror Lake

Mesa Creek

Pacific Crest Trail

Mesa Springs

N

Rock Mesa

0   0.5   1   1.5 miles

0   0.5   1   1.5 kilometers

The Wife

WILLAMETTE NATIONAL FOREST

Pacific Crest Trail

Le Conte Crater

DESCHUTES NATIONAL FOREST

Moraine Lake Trail

Wickiup Plain

The House Rock

Kaleetan Butte

Nash Lake Trail

Sisters Mirror Lake

Wickiup Plain Trail

Wickiup Plain Trail

Tyee Creek

Wickiup Plain Trail

Denude Lake

Kokostick Butte

Elk-Devils Trail

Blacktail Spring

to Bend

Koosah Mountain

Mirror Lake Trail

Pacific Crest Trail

Cascade Lakes Hwy.

Sink Creek

46

Even nicer is Lancelot Lake behind it, with several nice sites and an informal trail around it. Beyond that, I'll just say there are a few other nice lakes back there, all connected by informal trails, and I won't say much more because I want you to have your own adventure looking around back there—especially if you plan to camp in the area. (Or maybe I'm just trying to keep these secrets to myself!) Anyway, don't settle for Sisters Mirror Lake.

If you're feeling energetic, or if you're camping in the area and have some time to explore, consider putting in a few miles south on the PCT. It first passes Camelot Lake (apparently a Forest Service ranger thought the area resembled a jousting field, hence Camelot and Lancelot), and then it climbs 600 feet in 1.5 miles to the top of Koosah Mountain, where a sweeping view takes in South Sister, Broken Top, and Mount Bachelor.

Now, from the junction of Mirror Lakes Trail, which you came in on, the northbound PCT heads off to the east for a quarter mile to a junction with Wickiup Plains Trail, which here is signed for Moraine Lake. You could go east here to cut some distance off your hike (it's 4.5 boring miles back to the car that way), but the most

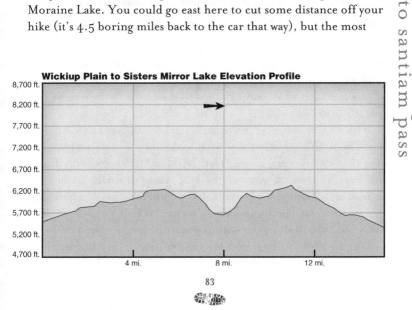

Wickiup Plain to Sisters Mirror Lake Elevation Profile

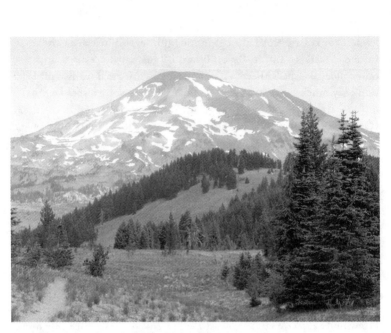

South Sister looms above the PCT in Wickiup Plain.

impressive scenery lies ahead on the PCT, which now turns northeast, rounds the eastern side of The House Rock, and then heads north and into the heart of Wickiup Plain, a pumice field thought to be about 20,000 years old.

With Le Conte Crater, Rock Mesa, and South Sister to your right, The Wife to your left, and what looks like the surface of the moon (but with flowers) at your feet, Wickiup Plain is indeed a dramatic stretch. After 1.6 miles on the PCT, come to a stark intersection with a trail signed for Devils Lake. We will take that one back, but I still recommend a bit more walking on the PCT. It's only 1.5 miles (with a small climb along the way) to where the trail crosses a beautiful creek on the edge of a large meadow, and from there it's just another mile (and down 300 feet) to the two forks of Mesa Creek, the second of which flows through an exquisite meadow with camping to the left—a fine place to spend the night or take an extended break.

Making your way back now, when you get to the junction in the middle of Wickiup Plain, turn left, following the sign for Devils Lake. Pass just south of Le Conte Crater (which you can scramble up for an interesting view) and, 1 mile later, turn right to follow a sign for Elk Lake. This is the Elk-Devils Trail, which you stick with for 3.1 miles (staying straight at 0.4 mile and turning right at 1.5 miles), all the way back to the original junction with Mirror Lakes Trail, at which point your car is 0.5 mile to your left.

For a longer and even more amazing loop, consider connecting this hike with either the Mink Lake Basin hike to the south (Hike 11, page 76), the Obsidian Loop (Hike 13, page 86), and Collier Glacier (Hike 14, page 92) walks to the north. Altogether these four hikes cover 31.5 miles of the PCT through this fantastic wilderness.

DIRECTIONS From Bend, go 30.1 miles west on Cascade Lakes Highway (FS 46) to the Mirror Lakes Trailhead.

PERMIT A Northwest Forest Pass is required.

GPS Trailhead Coordinates	12 Wickiup Plain to Sisters Mirror Lake
UTM Zone (WGS84)	10T
Easting	597631
Northing	4874430
Latitude	N44° 0.992'
Longitude	W121° 46.916'

13 Obsidian Loop

SCENERY: 🥾 🥾 🥾 🥾	HIKING TIME: *9 hours*
TRAIL CONDITION: 🥾 🥾 🥾	MAP: *Geo-Graphics Three Sisters Wilderness*
CHILDREN: 🥾	OUTSTANDING FEATURES: *Old-growth forest,*
DIFFICULTY: 🥾 🥾 🥾 🥾	*lava flows, babbling brooks, flower-filled meadows,*
SOLITUDE: 🥾 🥾	*soaring peaks, glaciers . . . basically, everything*
DISTANCE: *15.9 miles*	*that's good*

This hike approaches the same destination as the Lava Camp Lake to Collier Glacier View hike (Hike 14, page 92), but from the opposite direction. Where that hike explores lava fields and lakes, this one winds through meadows and over babbling brooks. It's also the perfect introduction to the heart of the Three Sisters Wilderness.

🥾🥾 When I close my eyes and think of beautiful places on the Oregon Pacific Crest Trail, my mind wanders to the Obsidian area. With alpine meadows, mountain views, crystalline waters, and soothing flowers, it is everything hiking should be. And that's why it's gotten so crowded that you need a permit to spend a night there; they are free but will be in great demand for summer weekends, so plan ahead.

Like so many good things in life, this section of the PCT also takes some work to attain. In this case, it's 5.4 miles from the trailhead to even reach the PCT, but those miles gain only 1,600 feet, and it's more than worth it.

From the trailhead, go 0.1 mile, and turn right onto Obsidian Trail (#3528). Pass a turnoff for Spring Lake at 0.9 mile, and then the grade mellows as you climb into cooler forest. At 1.75 miles, look for a lava flow on the right, climb near it for a mile, and then walk on it at 3 miles. Snake through the stone for almost a half mile, and emerge at a crossing of White Branch Creek and a junction with Glacier Way Trail (#4336). This is the way you'll come back on the loop, so for now turn right, following signs for Linton Meadows.

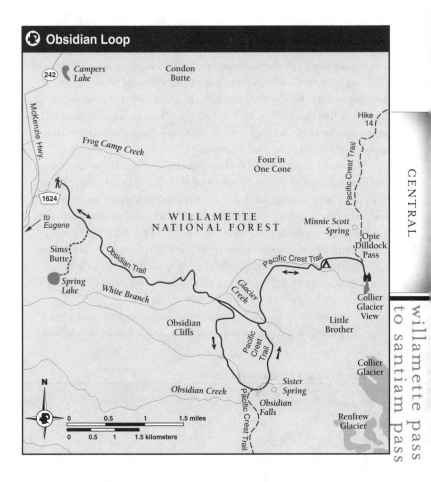

Obsidian Loop

242 Campers Lake

Condon Butte

McKenzie Hwy.

Frog Camp Creek

Four in One Cone

1624

to Eugene

WILLAMETTE NATIONAL FOREST

Minnie Scott Spring

Pacific Crest Trail

Opie Dilldock Pass

Obsidian Trail

Sims Butte

Spring Lake

White Branch

Glacier Creek

Pacific Crest Trail

Obsidian Cliffs

Little Brother

Collier Glacier View

Pacific Crest Trail

Collier Glacier

N

Obsidian Creek

Sister Spring

Obsidian Falls

Renfrew Glacier

0   0.5   1   1.5 miles

0   0.5   1   1.5 kilometers

Pacific Crest Trail

Hike 14

Over the next 2 miles, the forest opens up to reveal more and more meadows and views, and by the time you reach the PCT at 5.4 miles, you're at 6,400 feet elevation in a magical land of flowers and streams. You're also at a kind of decision point. I suggest a left-hand turn, but the area to the right is not exactly devoid of pleasures. In fact, my favorite spot in the wilderness, Linton Meadows, is about 3 miles to the south; it just happens not to be on the PCT. Still, consider camping a couple nights on this hike and exploring all around.

For now, turn left (north) onto the PCT, and in a minute or two pass lovely, 50-foot Obsidian Falls. And about that obsidian: it may look like black glass, and in fact it is. It's a particular kind of lava that, if conditions are right, cools into this shiny material. *It is profoundly illegal to take any of it home with you.*

Beyond Obsidian Falls, after passing under a large cliff on the right, look for Sister Spring and a series of small lakes. After topping a small ridge, look for a faint trail departing to the right and crossing a spring-fed creek; there's camping down there, and that trail goes up onto the snowfields of Middle Sister. Look for a campsite in the area (it must be at least 100 feet from trails and water), and go up that trail into the high country. Middle Sister is a challenging though nontechnical climb, but North Sister is a crumbly, technical, dangerous mess.

After a mile on the PCT, drop down to the upper crossing with the Glacier Way Trail, and a moment later take a bridge over Glacier

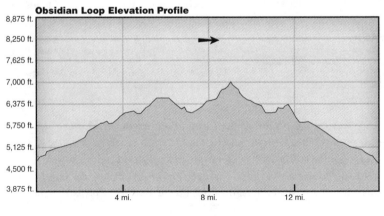

Obsidian Loop Elevation Profile

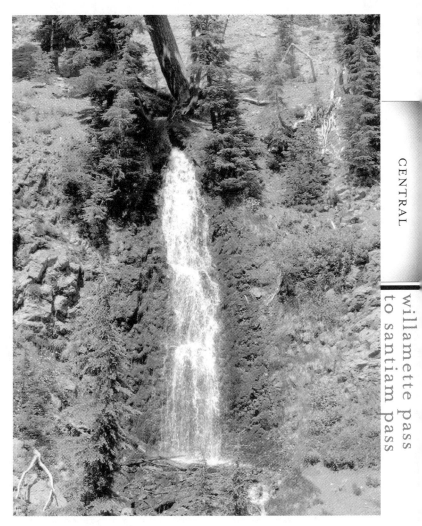

Obsidian Falls is on the PCT.

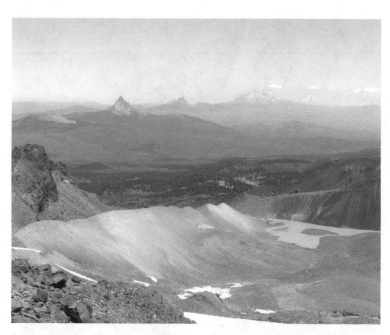

Looking north from the slopes of Middle Sister: Next up on the PCT (left to right) are Mount Washington, Three-Fingered Jack, Mount Jefferson, and Mount Hood.

Creek. This area (6.5 miles into your hike), known as Sunshine, is the heart of the area's alpine beauty and is generally closed to camping. If you want to cut a few miles off your loop, head back down the Glacier Way Trail here; otherwise, continue north on the PCT, cross the creek, and pass over a small ridge coming off of a peak called Little Brother. (The Three Sisters Wilderness also includes a Husband and Wife.)

One mile past Sunshine, the PCT reaches White Branch Creek and turns east to climb along it. A half mile up it crosses the creek at a place called Sawyer Bar; there's camping on the north side of the creek here. Now it's back onto the lava for 0.6 mile to Opie Dilldock

Pass, from where another climber's trail goes 0.4 mile out to Collier Glacier View—truly a seat at the foot of the mountains. (By the way, Opie Dilldock was a cartoon character from the early 20th century who always found a way out of seemingly impossible situations, and the rangers who scouted this tricky route in 1932 named the pass for him.)

To complete the loop, trace your steps back to Sunshine, and head steeply downhill on Glacier Way Trail. In 0.7 mile, reach the junction where the loop started, and from there follow Obsidian Trail 3.4 miles back to the car. You could also do a one-way car-shuttle hike and come out at the Lava Camp Trailhead by following the PCT 7 miles north from Dilldock Pass (the Lava Camp Lake to Collier Glacier hike, Hike 14, page 92) backward.

If you're *really* fired up, start with the Wickiup Plain hike (Hike 12, page 81), or even the Mink Lake Basin hike (Hike 11, page 76), and basically cross the whole wilderness. From the PCT near Elk Lake to McKenzie Pass—four hikes in this book—is 31.5 miles. It's amazing country; see as much of it as you can.

DIRECTIONS From Eugene, take OR 126 east for 56 miles to OR 242. Drive 16.7 miles up OR 242 to the Obsidian Trailhead.

PERMIT A Northwest Forest Pass is required for parking. A limited entry permit, available only via the Forest Service website, is required to spend the night within the Obsidian Permit Area. Reservations are $6 each and available for the entire season starting May 1.

GPS Trailhead Coordinates	13 Obsidian Loop
UTM Zone (WGS84)	10T
Easting	590266
Northing	4895225
Latitude	N44° 12.280'
Longitude	W121° 52.214'

14 Lava Camp Lake to Collier Glacier View

SCENERY: ✿ ✿ ✿ ✿	HIKING TIME: *10 hours*
TRAIL CONDITION: ✿ ✿ ✿ ✿	MAPS: *USFS* Three Sisters Wilderness; *most of the*
CHILDREN: ✿ ✿	*trail is also on Green Trails* Three Sisters.
DIFFICULTY: ✿ ✿ ✿	OUTSTANDING FEATURES: *Lava flows, alpine*
SOLITUDE: ✿ ✿ ✿	*meadows, long-distance vistas, and a seat at the foot of*
DISTANCE: *14.8 miles*	*a glacier-draped volcano*

Take a tour through about as much variety as a trail can offer: thick forest, lava flows, craters, sublime meadows, and a glacier. With numerous camping options spread along the trail, this can be a challenging day hike or a great, exploratory overnighter. In fact, since the south end of this hike is quite close to the north end of the Obsidian area hike (Hike 13, page 86), you could combine the two for a big Three Sisters adventure.

🏃🏃 Here's a bit of friendly advice: don't do this hike in July. I'm assuming you don't like mosquitoes, or heat, or potentially losing the trail in the snow. Wait until mid-August or so, when the flowers are peaking, and you won't have to deploy all your bug-avoidance maneuvers, gear, and substances.

Start behind the trail sign directing you to the Pacific Crest Trail. When you get to the PCT, turn left and begin climbing very gently on a wide path covered with needles and cones, through thick forest, and past the occasional meadow. In a little less than 1 mile, reach a junction for North and South Matthieu Lakes. This is the old Oregon Skyline Trail and is also an alternate path you could take to superior camping at the northern lake. To continue on the described route, stay on the PCT. At 2.1 miles the forest opens up a bit, allowing views of a ridge and lava flow ahead. The little saddle between the two is where you're headed.

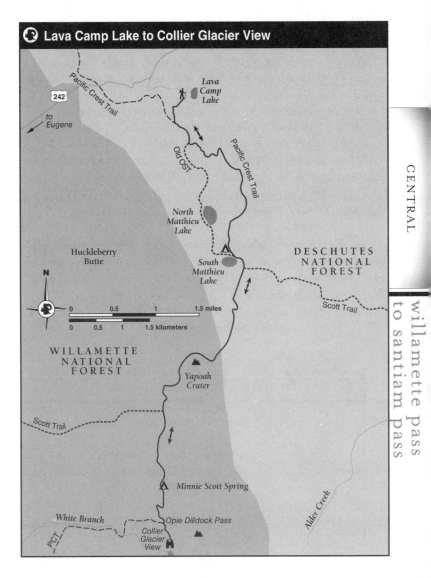

Lava Camp Lake to Collier Glacier View

to
Eugene

242

Pacific Crest Trail

Lava
Camp
Lake

Old OST

Pacific Crest Trail

North
Matthieu
Lake

Huckleberry
Butte

South
Matthieu
Lake

DESCHUTES
NATIONAL
FOREST

N

| 0 | 0.5 | 1 | 1.5 miles |

| 0 | 0.5 | 1 | 1.5 kilometers |

Scott Trail

WILLAMETTE
NATIONAL
FOREST

Yapoah
Crater

Scott Trail

Minnie Scott Spring

White Branch

Opie Dilldock Pass

PCT

Collier
Glacier
View

Alder Creek

93

As you continue, look for views on the right to Mount Washington and Three-Fingered Jack, the next two peaks north on the PCT. The little bump out in the lava flow is Little Belknap Crater, which is Hike 15 (page 98). Keep looking, and eventually Mount Jefferson comes into view on a clear day.

As you round a corner at 2.5 miles, catch your first view of North Sister, the most crumbly of the three peaks. You can also see North Matthieu Lake below you on the right.

Three miles out, arrive at South Matthieu Lake, where the alternate trail from below rejoins the PCT. At the far end of the lake, Scott Trail (#95) comes in from the left and runs with the PCT for the next 2.5 miles. There is decent camping here, but there are better spots ahead.

A half mile past the lake, get your first up-close encounter with lava, as the trail parallels a 400-year-old flow in an area that often has snow throughout July (we're above 6,000 feet in elevation now). You get to walk on the lava for a bit (trust me, it gets hot in July) and find yourself walking toward the source of all this rock: Yapoah Crater, a reddish cone ahead and on the left.

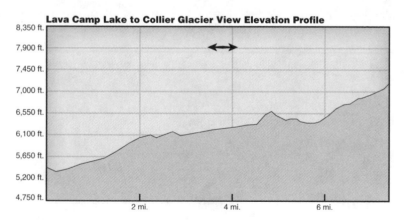

Lava Camp Lake to Collier Glacier View Elevation Profile

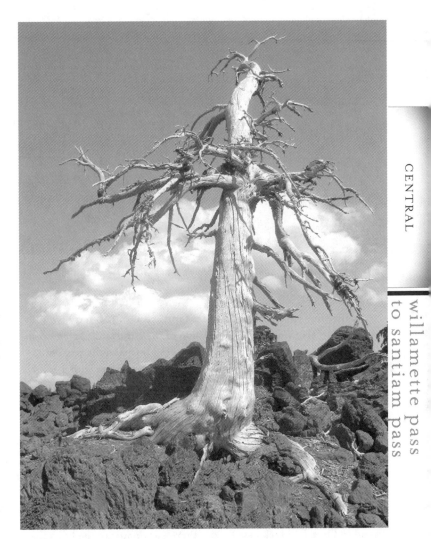

A hardy, even if dead, tree out in the lava fields near Yapoah Crater

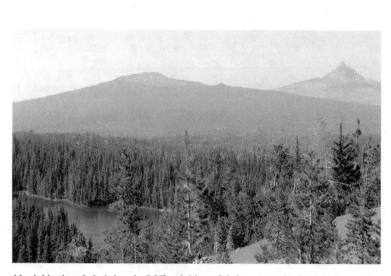

North Matthieu Lake below the PCT with Mount Washington in the distance

By the time you've put in 5 miles (and are at 6,500 feet), you'll have climbed around the southwest side of the cone and started down into lovely, greener country. The Scott Trail leaves to the west, at 5.5 miles, and just 0.1 mile later you enter a broad meadow with a creek and a million flowers.

Now we'll start our climb for the day—there had to be a climb, right? Look for Mount Adams, in the distance on your right, and flat-topped (and much smaller) Coffin Mountain on the left, which is way over by Detroit Lake. One mile past Scott Trail's departure (and 400 feet above it), come to Minnie Scott Spring, named for the niece of Felix Scott, the trail's namesake. There's space for one or two tents on some flat ground west of the spring—no permits necessary.

Keep climbing, and within another 0.6 mile (and 200 feet) ascend to Opie Dilldock Pass—and if there's any name in the book that needs explaining, it's Opie Dilldock. The story goes like this: In 1932, a couple of Forest Service guys were looking for a way down into the White Branch canyon (just a mile south of here the PCT crosses White Branch). When they finally found the right spot, they named it for Opie Dilldock, an early 20th-century comic book character who always found a way out of tough situations. So there you have it.

From the pass, the PCT continues west, onto the lava, and eventually to the sublime Obsidian special permit area (see Hike 13, page 86). For now, take the mountaineers' trail south from the 6,800-foot pass to climb to the southern edge of the cone (about 300 feet up in 0.3 mile) and witness a spectacular view to Collier Glacier on the west side of North Sister. Also prominent here, really for the first time in your hike, is the north side of Middle Sister.

It's not too much more work (without your heavy pack, anyway) to explore this area further, aiming for either the saddle between Middle and North Sisters or the summit of Middle Sister itself. Climber trails abound and are generally marked with rock cairns. Even if you pass on the climbing, you can't do much better than hanging out in this area for a little while.

DIRECTIONS From Sisters, drive 14 miles west on OR 242 to the turnoff for Lava Camp Lake. Turn left, and in 0.3 mile stay right for the trailhead, rather than left for the campground. A Northwest Forest Pass is required, and there are no facilities at the trailhead.

PERMIT A Northwest Forest Pass is required.

GPS Trailhead Coordinates	14 Lava Camp Lake to Collier Glacier View
UTM Zone (WGS84)	10T
Easting	596964
Northing	4901299
Latitude	N44° 15.508'
Longitude	W121° 47.118'

15 Little Belknap Crater

SCENERY: ✿ ✿ ✿
TRAIL CONDITION: ✿ ✿
CHILDREN: ✿ ✿ ✿
DIFFICULTY: ✿ ✿
SOLITUDE: ✿ ✿ ✿

DISTANCE: *4.8 miles*
HIKING TIME: *2½ hours*
MAP: *Green Trails* Three Fingered Jack
OUTSTANDING FEATURES: *Lava flows and mountain views*

This little leg stretcher is absolutely unlike any other hike on the Oregon Pacific Crest Trail—or any other section of it, for that matter. For all but a few minutes, the trail here is on lava, and in fact it goes up the flow to its origin, a small crater with a big view. It's a good one for kids, but not for lightweight shoes or folks with knee problems.

🚶🚶 All the lava around McKenzie Pass is relatively new—geologically speaking. The oldest you'll walk on here is 3,000 years old at most. Very few plants have managed to colonize it; save this one for a cloudy day or the autumn, when temperatures are less brutal. PCT thru-hikers tend to come through here in August and have been known to hike this hot, dry section at night.

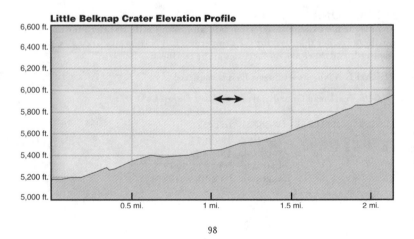

Little Belknap Crater Elevation Profile

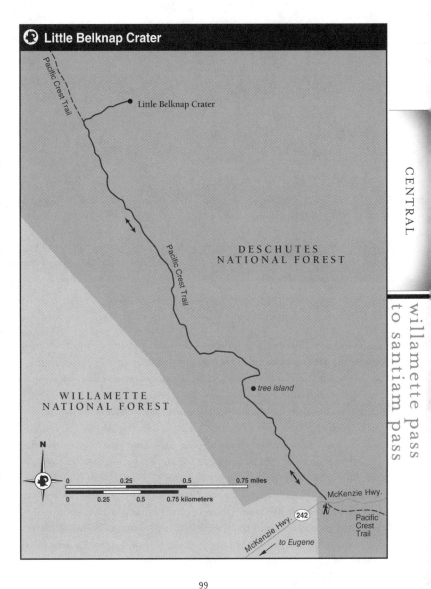

Little Belknap Crater

Little Belknap Crater

Pacific Crest Trail

Pacific Crest Trail

DESCHUTES
NATIONAL FOREST

WILLAMETTE
NATIONAL FOREST

• *tree island*

N

| 0 | 0.25 | 0.5 | 0.75 miles |

| 0 | 0.25 | 0.5 | 0.75 kilometers |

McKenzie Hwy.

Pacific
Crest
Trail

McKenzie Hwy. (242)

← *to Eugene*

willamette pass
to santiam pass

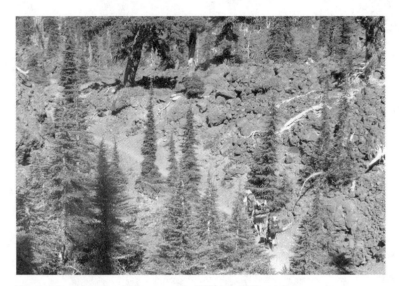

Winding through lava and rare trees on the PCT near McKenzie Pass

From the trailhead, start out in a thin pine forest, and follow the trail north toward a clump of trees about 0.3 mile ahead. This "island" of trees was missed by the latest lava flow, rather like an eddy in a river. The trail swings to the right of these trees, crosses the lava "current" for 100 yards, and then heads for a second island of trees. Note, as you wrap around the west side of this island, that the south side, which catches most of the summer sun, is quite a bit drier than the north side.

When you leave the trees behind for good, you've gone 0.8 mile, and if the immediate scenery is getting old, you can at least look back for nice views of Middle and North Sisters and Black Crater, as well as up ahead to reddish Belknap Crater, your destination's big brother.

The grade gets a little steep during this 1.5-mile walk, but it never gets intense. Then, just before the trail's high point, a rock cairn marks the side trail to the crater. Once you're on this ridge trail, you can look out to the north and see Mount Washington, which is what's left of a volcano after a series of glaciers got through with it.

The only really steep section of this hike is at the very end, where you might occasionally have to scramble a bit. In fact, this whole trail would be rough on a pair of sneakers, so wear some stiff-soled boots.

From the top, your view extends from the rolling lava fields at your feet south to North and Middle Sisters, and of course north to Mount Washington. Middle Sister is on the right, and the glacier on the left side of it is the Collier Glacier. The Lava Camp Lake to Collier Glacier View hike (Hike 14, page 92), which starts almost directly across the highway, goes to a wonderful viewpoint of that glacier.

Little Belknap might strike you as an odd-looking volcano, but in fact it's what's known as a shield volcano—so called because it's said to resemble a warrior's shield. A shield volcano is formed by eruptions of highly liquid lava; since it flows so easily, it makes a long, broad slope like the one you just hiked up, rather than piling up steeply. Three-Fingered Jack and Mount Thielsen are also (highly eroded) shield volcanoes.

DIRECTIONS From Sisters, drive 15 miles west on OR 242 to McKenzie Pass. A half mile west of the Dee Wright Observatory at the pass, turn right into the parking lot at a brown hiker sign.

PERMIT A Northwest Forest Pass is required.

GPS Trailhead Coordinates	15 Little Belknap Crater
UTM Zone (WGS84)	10T
Easting	595049
Northing	4901447
Latitude	N44° 15.604'
Longitude	W121° 48.555'

16 Three-Fingered Jack

SCENERY: ⭐ ⭐ ⭐
TRAIL CONDITION: ⭐ ⭐ ⭐
CHILDREN: ⭐ ⭐
DIFFICULTY: ⭐ ⭐
SOLITUDE: ⭐ ⭐ ⭐ ⭐
DISTANCE: 9.5 miles

HIKING TIME: *6 hours*
MAP: *Green Trails* Three Fingered Jack
OUTSTANDING FEATURES: *A ghostly postfire landscape, two mountain lakes, a soaring mountain viewpoint, and a wonderful meadow*

Most day hikers never make it above Canyon Creek Meadows. And Pacific Crest Trail thru-hikers, hustling between Santiam Pass and the Mount Jefferson Wilderness, might not take much notice of poor, broken-down old Three-Fingered Jack. But it's a fascinating mountain, and this is your chance to get up close and personal with it—and also to see what a forest looks like after a fire, visit (and possibly camp at) two fine lakes, and stroll through a couple of wonderful meadows.

🚶🚶 If you get to the Jack Lake Trailhead and see two dozen cars, don't fret; very few of them are going where you're headed. Most of them are doing a loop through Canyon Creek Meadows, which you will see. Others are camping at Wasco Lake, which you will also see. But very few of them are climbing to the shoulder of Three-Fingered Jack, where you're going, for two simple reasons: they don't know about it, and there's a hill on the way.

Start by walking toward Jack Lake and following a trail around its right side. You are in a lovely, dry forest typical of those on the east side of the Cascades, and if it's sunny out, you'll feel it. Through the trees to the left, you can make out Three-Fingered Jack (allegedly named for a three-fingered trapper who lived in the area); your destination is just out of sight to the right of the summit.

Start climbing slowly through a forest that burned in the 2003 B&B Fire, which started as two fires, combined into one near this area, and swept through some 91,000 acres. But as you'll see during your

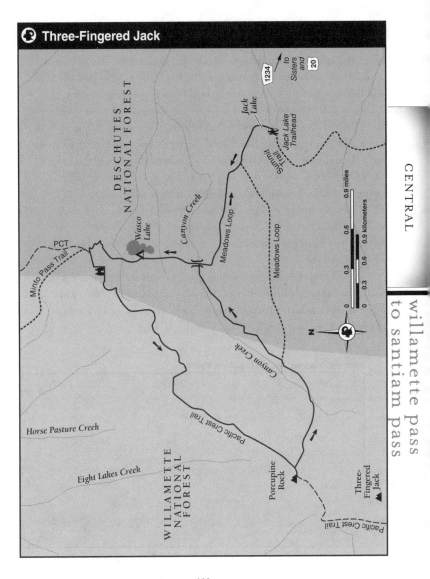

walk, whole patches of forest were untouched, even though others were decimated. In some places, you can find patches of green in heavily scorched areas but also brown scorched spots in green areas. I spoke with a trail maintenance volunteer for this section, who said the area will have a lot more blown-down dead trees in coming winters.

At a little less than a half mile, reach the intersection where the Canyon Creek Meadows Loop begins. This wildly popular walk has an interesting twist: the Forest Service wants the traffic to go in a clockwise loop from this point. So, technically, by turning right toward Wasco Lake, we're going the wrong way, but since we're not going to the meadows (yet), it doesn't matter (for now).

Keep walking through various degrees of fire damage and, a half mile past the junction, pass an impressive glacial erratic boulder on the left—so called because it was deposited here thousands of years ago by a glacier.

At 1.6 miles, you come to a second junction, the return of the Canyon Creek Meadows Loop. Stay right, again for Wasco Lake, and a few moments later, ford Canyon Creek between two waterfalls. You might get your feet wet here early in the season.

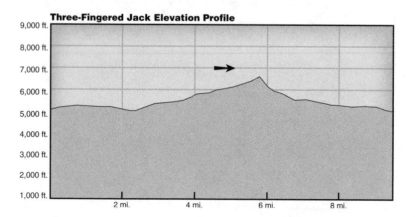

Three-Fingered Jack Elevation Profile

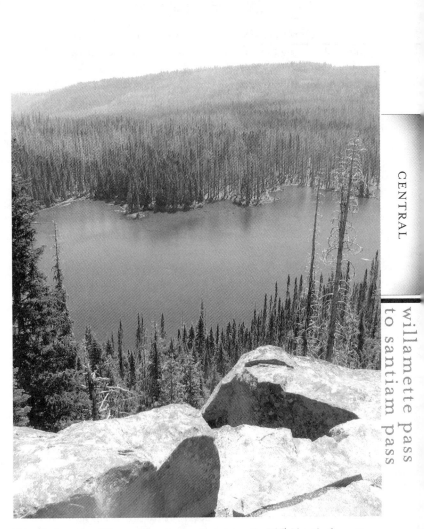

Wasco Lake, with excellent camping, from a viewpoint on the PCT: Note the fire patterns in the forest.

When you come to Wasco Lake a half mile later, there are a series of campsites along the left-hand shore, most of them in areas that burned in 2003. The good (unburned) sites are at the far end of the lake, right where you turn left (and way up) on Trail 4015, which is labeled here as PCNST, or Pacific Crest National Scenic Trail—its official name. This trail picks up 200 feet in a fun quarter mile and deposits you onto the PCT at Minto Pass.

Follow the PCT to your left, which is southwest, toward Three-Fingered Jack, and in a few minutes you are rewarded with a panoramic view back toward Black Butte in the distance and Wasco Lake in the foreground—along with a whole bunch of fire damage. Again, note how the fire skipped patches of forest. Take a little break here, because the next few miles pick up a thousand feet of elevation.

Climb for a little more than 2 miles to a minor saddle, where you cross over onto the east side of the ridge—a nice spot, but not the top. That's a half mile up, at the top of four switchbacks out on the open, rocky slope east of Porcupine Rock. From the top, at 6,500 feet, enjoy a grand view of upper Canyon Creek Meadows and the multicolored, many layered north face of Three-Fingered Jack, whose summit is 1,300 messy, rocky feet above you. It is, in fact, the remnants of an ancient volcano. Another interesting feature is to your left: note how one side of Porcupine Rock burned and the other one didn't.

You could go back the way you came, but let's have a little adventure. Start back down the switchbacks and, just past the fourth one, look for a marginal trail plunging down to the right. Take it. It will be clear and easy to follow for a while and then will seem to disappear into an area of large boulders; find it again toward the right.

Next comes a sloping, open hillside where you again stay right—but, at this point, the main thing is don't go too far left—and have faith. As the trail's steepness mellows out (the first half mile loses 700 feet!), simply head for the sound of water, and when in doubt, aim for a notch on the left side of Three-Fingered Jack. There's a lake up there, and you will cross the creek flowing out of it. Also, look for a trail that comes out of woods at the far end of the meadow. Cross Canyon Creek where you can, then head for that trail.

This trail leads over a small rise, down through a lovely, narrow meadow, through a fine stand of mountain hemlock, and finally to the outer edge of the one-way meadows loop—a total drop of 1,000 feet in 1.5 miles. Here again are the one-way hiking trails. Going the "correct" way, which is left, makes for a longer hike but will take you by some beaver-worked trees; look for them on your left. You'll go 0.7 mile along Canyon Creek, which brings you back to your original trail, where you turn right and go 1.4 miles to the car; follow the signs for the Jack Lake Trailhead.

On the drive out, if your feet are sore, stop and soak them in Jack Creek—or, I should say, see if you can soak your feet in Jack Creek. It is cold! And it is, therefore, exactly what you'll want. You might even take a short trail to visit the charming area around the head of Jack Spring; turn right at the creek and go a short way up FS 400 to find the trail in a small campground.

DIRECTIONS From Sisters, go 12.4 miles northwest on US 20, and turn north onto FS 12. Follow FS 12 for 4.5 miles, then go 1.7 miles north on FS 1230. Turn left (west) on FS 1234, which is pretty wash-boarded, and follow it 6.2 winding, bumpy miles to the trailhead at the end of the road.

PERMIT A Northwest Forest Pass is required.

GPS Trailhead Coordinates	16 Three-Fingered Jack
UTM Zone (WGS84)	10T
Easting	595872
Northing	4927222
Latitude	N44° 29.517'
Longitude	W121° 47.652'

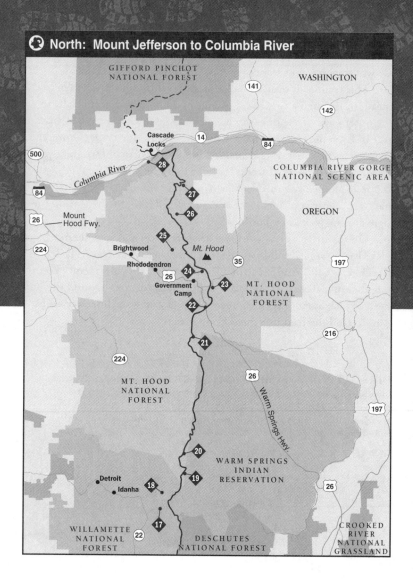

GIFFORD PINCHOT
NATIONAL FOREST

WASHINGTON

141

142

500

84

Cascade
Locks

14

84

Columbia River

28

COLUMBIA RIVER GORGE
NATIONAL SCENIC AREA

OREGON

26

Mount
Hood Fwy.

27

26

224

26

25

Brightwood

Rhododendron

26

24

Mt. Hood

35

197

23

MT. HOOD
NATIONAL
FOREST

Government
Camp

22

216

21

224

MT. HOOD
NATIONAL
FOREST

26

Warm Springs Hwy.

197

20

WARM SPRINGS
INDIAN
RESERVATION

Detroit

Idanha

18

19

26

17

WILLAMETTE
NATIONAL
FOREST

22

DESCHUTES
NATIONAL FOREST

CROOKED
RIVER
NATIONAL
GRASSLAND

3

NORTH

Mount Jefferson to
Columbia River

17 Pamelia Lake to Shale Lake Loop (*page 110*)

18 Jefferson Park (*page 116*)

19 Breitenbush Lake to Park Butte (*page 122*)

20 Olallie Lake to Upper Lake (*page 129*)

21 Little Crater Lake to Timothy Lake (*page 135*)

22 Twin Lakes Loop (*page 140*)

23 Barlow Pass to Timberline Lodge (*page 145*)

24 Timberline Lodge to Paradise Park (*page 150*)

25 Ramona Falls to Sandy River Loop (*page 158*)

26 Lost Lake to Buck Peak (*page 166*)

27 Chinidere Mountain (*page 172*)

28 Eagle Creek to Benson Plateau Loop (*page 178*)

17 Pamelia Lake to Shale Lake Loop

SCENERY: ✿ ✿ ✿ ✿	HIKING TIME: *10 hours*
TRAIL CONDITION: ✿ ✿ ✿	MAP: *Green Trails* Mt. Jefferson *or*
CHILDREN: ✿ ✿	USFS Mt. Jefferson Wilderness
DIFFICULTY: ✿ ✿ ✿	OUTSTANDING FEATURES: *Several beautiful*
SOLITUDE: ✿ ✿	*lakes, remnants of a dramatic rockslide, mountains*
DISTANCE: *19 miles*	*views, and a fascinating watershed*

This epic loop on the south side of Mount Jefferson takes in lakes, forest, sweeping views, alpine wonderlands, and some of the most scenic campsites you'll find anywhere. Note that if you want to camp at Pamelia Lake, you have to get a permit online and stick to designated sites.

🚶🚶 If you're looking for a two- or three-day loop to introduce you to a less-crowded corner of wilderness, try this one. You can also do variations on this, keeping it to as little as 4.5 miles (just to see Pamelia Lake) or using it as a starting point for exploring the southern Mount Jefferson Wilderness. If nothing else, the area around Shale Lake is worth exploring as a kind of less-crowded version of Jefferson Park, on the mountain's north side.

From the trailhead, start up a wide, barely climbing forest path along Pamelia Creek, named after a girl on an 1879 exploration party for her "unfailing cheerfulness." It would be hard not to be cheerful in a place like this. Around the 2-mile mark, look for a faint trail leading to the right to Flapper Spring, the outlet creek of Pamelia Lake that was buried long ago by a rockslide (more on this later).

At 2.2 miles, reach a trail junction at the lake's northern edge. You can explore for a while, if you'd like, but by late summer, this lake isn't much to look at. Take the left (uphill) trail at this junction,

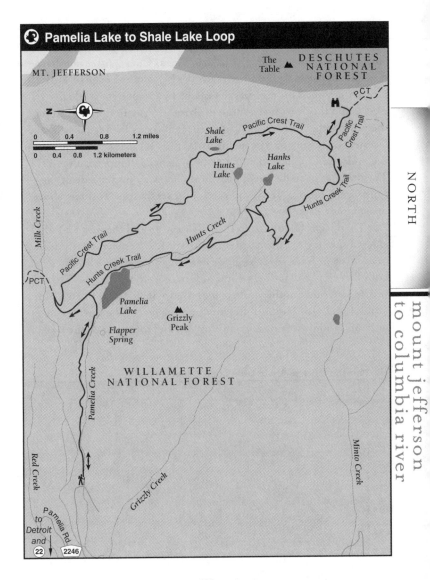

MT. JEFFERSON

The Table ▲

DESCHUTES NATIONAL FOREST

PCT

N

0   0.4   0.8   1.2 miles
0   0.4   0.8   1.2 kilometers

Shale Lake

Pacific Crest Trail

Hanks Lake

Pacific Crest Trail

Hunts Lake

Milk Creek

Pacific Crest Trail

Hunts Creek Trail

Hunts Creek

Hunts Creek Trail

PCT

Pamelia Lake

Grizzly Peak ▲

Flapper Spring

Pamelia Creek

WILLAMETTE NATIONAL FOREST

Red Creek

to Detroit and
22   2246

Pamelia Rd.

Grizzly Creek

Minto Creek

mount jefferson to columbia river

staying on Trail 3439 toward the Pacific Crest Trail. In 0.3 mile turn left at the junction of Trail 3440. (Turning right here leads along the east side of Pamelia Lake to Hunts Cove.) After another 0.4 mile of gradual climbing, reach the PCT on the edge of Milk Creek Canyon. This area was devastated by a major rockslide in 2007, and this rerouted section explains why the first bit of trail on the north side of the creek is so steep. It also gets hit regularly by avalanches, including one in spring 2011. Fifty yards left of the junction is a multi-ton boulder that the 2007 avalanche dumped on the PCT. The trail has been diverted to avoid it. Standing on the side of the Milk Creek canyon, see if you can spot scars on trees 100 feet above the summer water level.

Turn right (south) onto the PCT, and round the west end of a ridge. Catching occasional views south toward Pamelia Lake, put in 3 unexciting miles before the grade lets up, and there are fine views of both Pamelia Lake far below and of Grizzly Peak opposite. The trail swings east, and another mile brings you to Shale Lake, in an alpine wonderland with Mount Jefferson looming just to the north. At 6.9 miles in, and with fantastic camping east and southeast of the lake,

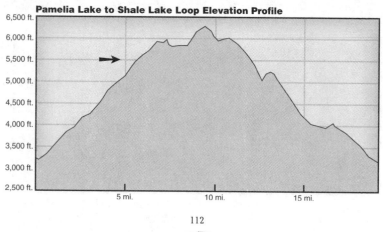

Pamelia Lake to Shale Lake Loop Elevation Profile

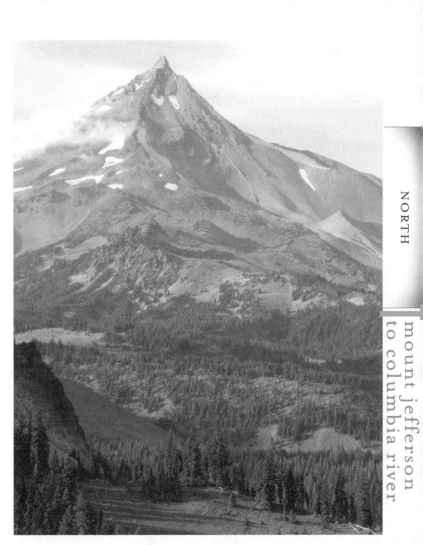

The awesome south side of Mount Jefferson, with The Table in the foreground, from the PCT just south of Hunts Cove

this is a fine place to spend at least one night. There are numerous other lakes to check out, and you might even find a climber's trail heading above timberline toward the southwest side of Jefferson. A permit is required to camp at these lakes.

South of Shale Lake, the PCT stays flat for 0.3 mile before dropping slightly toward Hunts Cove, a dramatic bowl with two major lakes. The trail traverses the east side of the cove, passing under the Cathedral Rocks, and after 1.8 miles reaches a saddle and junction with Hunts Creek Trail (#3440). A less-developed trail plunges into Hunts Cove (#3430), but it's steep and unnecessary; by following #3440 you can get to the same place. Both of these trails are infrequently maintained.

The main hike heads west here, but before that, it's worth making a 1.5-mile round-trip excursion south on the PCT to an amazing viewpoint that includes The Table and its volcanic surroundings— and, of course, Jefferson. This spot may be the best view of Oregon's second-highest peak.

From back at the saddle, head west now on Hunts Creek Trail to gradually descend along 1.6 miles to a junction with Trail 3493, which takes off south for Lake of the Woods and, eventually, Marion Lake. Now Trail 3440 plunges down a series of switchbacks to another junction, this one at the mouth of Hunts Cove. It's certainly worth exploring (or camping in) the cove; from here, Hanks Lake is 0.5 mile up this trail, and Hunts Lake is another 0.4 mile past that. There are fine campsites at both lakes, though Hunts gets less traffic. Camping at either requires a permit.

Heading downhill from this junction, the Hunts Creek Trail now enters a flowery, water-filled valley that feeds into Pamelia Lake. There's an amazing amount of water headed down these hills, which means it can get muggy in the summer, but there are also plenty of chances to cool off. Cross Hunts Creek 2 miles down (there's no bridge and you might have to wade), and soon you are at the upper end of Pamelia Lake. Working your way along the shoreline, you might notice that even with all that water flowing into the lake, there's no apparent outlet. That's because it was buried by that slide and now flows mostly underground—hence, the name "Flapper Spring."

It's 1.3 miles from the Hunts Creek crossing to the junction where this whole loop started, and from there an easy 2.2 miles back to the trailhead. And then, some 17 miles and 4,000 feet of gain later in your car, you can go to Detroit and get a burger.

DIRECTIONS From Detroit, head east on OR 22 for 12 miles, and turn left (east) onto Pamelia Rd. (FS 2246). The trailhead is at the end of this road, 3.7 miles ahead. The last 400 yards of road are unpaved.

PERMIT A Northwest Forest Pass is required for parking. A limited entry permit, available only via the Forest Service website, is required for access to the area mentioned in this description including Hunts Cove and Shale Lake. Reservations are $6 each and available for the entire season starting May 1.

GPS Trailhead Coordinates	17 Pamelia Lake to Shale Lake Loop
UTM Zone (WGS84)	10T
Easting	587929
Northing	4945750
Latitude	N44° 39.584'
Longitude	W121° 53.455'

18 Jefferson Park

SCENERY: ⛺ ⛺ ⛺ ⛺	HIKING TIME: *9 hours*
TRAIL CONDITION: ⛺ ⛺ ⛺	MAP: *Green Trails* Mount Jefferson *or*
CHILDREN: ⛺ ⛺	*Geo-Graphics* Mount Jefferson Wilderness
DIFFICULTY: ⛺ ⛺ ⛺	OUTSTANDING FEATURES: *Old-growth forest,*
SOLITUDE: ⛺	*alpine meadows, rushing creeks, and a flower-filled*
DISTANCE: *14.9 miles*	*wonderland at the base of Oregon's second-highest peak*

Some of my finest backpacking nights have been spent in Jefferson Park, with its lakes, meadows, flowers, and front-row view of Mount Jefferson. Two notes to consider though: it gets crowded on weekends, and before August, you'll be in a fog of mosquitoes.

Some day fairly soon, the Forest Service will probably have to limit access to Jefferson Park, as it does with the Obsidian area in the Three Sisters Wilderness. It's one of those ironies of the mountains: The places that are beautiful and easy to get to eventually get overused. What can you do? Go during the week, especially after Labor Day, and don't go tramping around on the meadows. As you'll see, there are plenty of trails to use.

From the trailhead, start a wonderfully gradual climb: about 1,500 feet in 2.6 miles. Though you can't see any mountains yet, the view is nonetheless sublime as you switchback up through a magnificent mid-elevation old-growth fir forest. After 1.5 miles of this mellow splendor, reach a trail intersection and turn right to stay on Jefferson Park Trail, #3429.

Keep climbing for another mile, passing a clearing with a view back down the valley of Whitewater Creek, and then round the southern end of a ridge. One mile from the junction, pass through a saddle, and head for the southern edge of the Sentinel Hills, which you traverse with an ever-improving view of Mount Jefferson ahead.

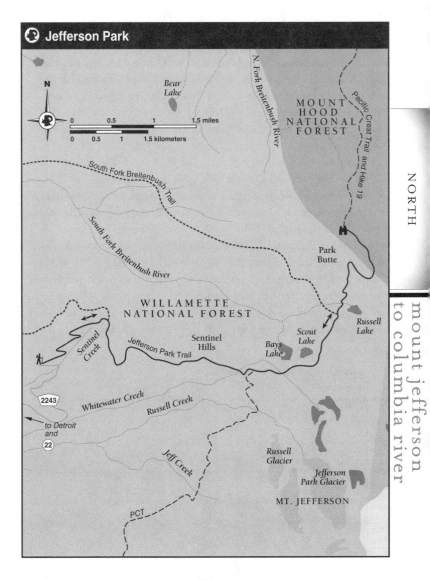

Jefferson Park

Bear Lake

N. Fork Breitenbush River

MOUNT HOOD NATIONAL FOREST

Pacific Crest Trail and Hike 19

N

0   0.5   1   1.5 miles

0   0.5   1   1.5 kilometers

South Fork Breitenbush Trail

South Fork Breitenbush River

Park Butte

WILLAMETTE NATIONAL FOREST

Russell Lake

Scout Lake

Sentinel Hills

Bays Lake

Sentinel Creek

Jefferson Park Trail

2243

Whitewater Creek

Russell Creek

to Detroit and 22

Jeff Creek

Russell Glacier

Jefferson Park Glacier

PCT

MT. JEFFERSON

mount jefferson to columbia river

After 1.3 flat miles, cross Whitewater Creek and climb slightly for a quarter mile to the PCT, which to the south traverses Jefferson's west side on a 9-mile stretch from Shale Lake. As you can see, it's possible (and recommended) to connect this hike with the Pamelia Lake to Shale Lake Loop (Hike 17, page 110) or the Breitenbush Lake to Park Butte hike (Hike 19, page 122), which lies north of here. The walk from Pamelia Lake to Breitenbush Lake on the PCT is about 20 miles.

For now, though, turn left onto the PCT and follow its northbound route gently uphill for a mile—and start getting used to all these flowers and meadows. In August, when the flowers are in full bloom, it's tough to keep up a reasonable pace with all the gawking. Climb a final hill, swing around to the north, and welcome to Jefferson Park.

The first thing you'll notice is that there are a lot of trails. Few of them are official, however. The unfortunate reality is that so many people come up here that there aren't enough designated campsites for everyone (hence the plans for permits); for now people just wander all over the place, looking for places to camp. Signs at the trailhead (and the staff at the Detroit Ranger Station) will tell you where

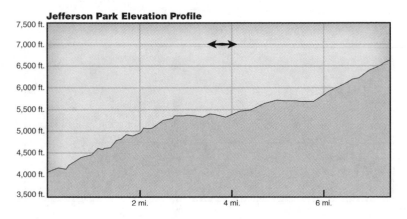

Jefferson Park Elevation Profile

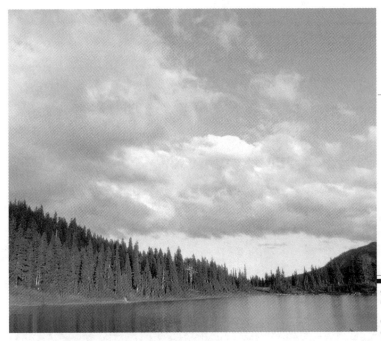

The PCT passes several nice campsites along Russell Lake in Jefferson Park.

camping is legitimate, but the general rule of thumb is that if you're within 250 feet of a lake and don't see a campsite sign with a triangle, don't camp there. Fires are prohibited throughout Jefferson Park.

Still, plan to spend a night. Scout Lake, the first big one on the left, is quite popular. My personal favorite sites are on the far side of Bays Lake, west of Scout. Beautiful Russell Lake, at the far end, has at least three designated sites.

Once you've found a site or rested from the climb up, you have three general options: explore the lake areas, look for a climber's trail

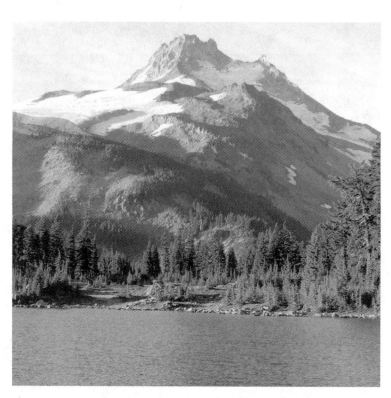

The north side of Mount Jefferson from Russell Lake, just off the PCT in Jefferson Park. Jefferson Park Glacier is on the left.

up onto the mountain that starts east of where you entered the basin, or follow the PCT across it and up to the top of Park Butte. (The mileage for this hike is figured as a round-trip to the butte.)

Along the way to the butte, you cross the South Fork Breitenbush River and its adjacent trail (#3375). If you're looking for a pleasant way out of the wilderness, take this trail; it leads about 8.5 miles down to another trail that leads 2.5 more miles to Breitenbush Hot

Springs. If you're looking for a good campsite, check about 50 yards past the (tiny) river.

Beyond this junction, the PCT starts to climb out of Jefferson Park, a 2-mile, 1,110-foot ascent to a spectacular vista point of Jefferson Park, Mount Jefferson, Mount Hood, and much of its namesake national forest to the north. This spot is also the southernmost point of the Breitenbush Lake to Park Butte hike (Hike 19, page 122).

A social trail leads west, then south, along the ridge, first past the official summit at 7,018 feet, and then to the 6,851-foot hill officially called Park Butte. There's a tremendous view of the lakes in Jefferson Park from out there, but this 0.7-mile trail is not for kids or anybody afraid of heights.

If you're wondering about some of the names, Mount Jefferson is one of the few things around with a name bestowed by Lewis and Clark's Corps of Discovery; they saw it on March 30, 1806, from a spot near Portland's location and named it for the president who sent them west. Breitenbush (actually Breitenbusher) was the name of an early pioneer.

DIRECTIONS From Detroit, go east on OR 22 for 10 miles and turn north onto Whitewater Rd., which is also marked as FS 2243. The trailhead is 7.4 miles ahead, at the end of the road.

PERMIT A Northwest Forest Pass is required.

GPS Trailhead Coordinates	18 Jefferson Park
UTM Zone (WGS84)	10T
Easting	589098
Northing	4950990
Latitude	N44° 42.405'
Longitude	W121° 52.515'

19 Breitenbush Lake to Park Butte

SCENERY: ⛺ ⛺ ⛺ ⛺	HIKING TIME: *4 hours*
TRAIL CONDITION: ⛺ ⛺ ⛺	MAP: *Green Trails* Mt. Jefferson *or*
CHILDREN: ⛺	*USFS* Mt. Jefferson Wilderness
DIFFICULTY: ⛺ ⛺ ⛺	OUTSTANDING FEATURES: *Meadows, rock*
SOLITUDE: ⛺ ⛺	*fields, late summer snow, and a monster mountain*
DISTANCE: *7 miles*	*viewpoint*

This classic walk can be a moderately challenging day hike, an easy overnight hike, or part of a two- or three-day exploration of the area north of Mount Jefferson. If nothing else, extend it down into Jefferson Park and consider combining it with the Jefferson Park hike (Hike 18, page 116). You can't find a dull hike in this part of the world!

🚶 Hikers are funny folks sometimes. Everybody knows about Jefferson Park, and just about everybody comes at it from a trailhead down near Santiam Pass—and, faithful guide that I am, I describe that hike elsewhere in this book (Hike 18). The Jefferson Park hike is easier, 'tis true. But this hike, to a ridge that looms 1,200 feet above Jefferson Park, is shorter, more scenic, and less traveled. How funny—and fortunate for us. The price you pay is mostly the drive to the trailhead (see directions for details).

But before we start walking, let's give credit to the hardworking folks who maintain this section of trail: the West Cascade Chapter of Backcountry Horsemen of Oregon. The trail north of here is handled by, believe it or not, a group called the Oregon Mule Skinners. All this is on behalf of the Mount Hood Chapter of the Pacific Crest Trail Association. Yay trail workers!

Begin the hike by following a short spur trail southwest from the parking lot to the PCT. Then turn left in a series of meadows filled with lupines, daisies, and clouds of migratory monarch butterflies— all this in August, which is, not only the best time to do this hike, but

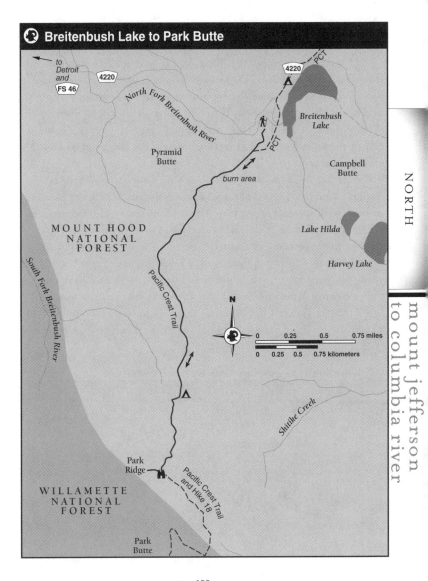

to
Detroit
and
FS 46

4220

North Fork Breitenbush River

4220

PCT

Breitenbush
Lake

PCT

Pyramid
Butte

burn area

Campbell
Butte

MOUNT HOOD
NATIONAL
FOREST

Lake Hilda

South Fork Breitenbush River

Pacific Crest Trail

Harvey Lake

N

0   0.25   0.5   0.75 miles

0   0.25   0.5   0.75 kilometers

Shitike Creek

Park
Ridge

Pacific Crest Trail
and Hike 18

WILLAMETTE
NATIONAL
FOREST

Park
Butte

NORTH

mount jefferson
to columbia river

also the first month when you won't have to deal with tons of snow and hordes of mosquitoes.

After 0.6 mile of easy strolling, you'll be in an area that burned intensely a few years ago. There used to be a bridge over a creekbed here; now the trail crosses below, and the charred remnants of the bridge are visible in the bed. It's fascinating, as always, to note how the fire destroyed some areas and skipped others. At times, from this trail, you can make out the exact lines where the fire stopped and the greenery remains.

At 0.7 mile, approach a rockslide with a sweeping view north. Around 2 miles out, you enter an area that typically exhibits patches of snow well into July, even into August. The snowy ground inspires hikers to create multiple trails as alternates to the snowfields; just stay on the biggest one and watch for rock cairns or pieces of wood conspicuously sticking up out of rock piles. And remember, if you're going up, you're going the right way. The ridge you can make out just to the right of Mount Jefferson, up ahead, is your destination.

At 2.7 miles (and 6,400 feet), there's a small lake on the left and a campsite on the right with a metal fire ring. If you're looking for

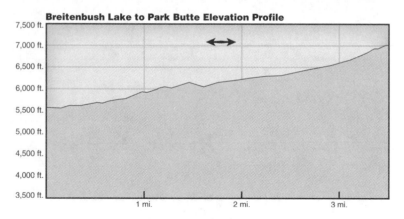

Breitenbush Lake to Park Butte Elevation Profile

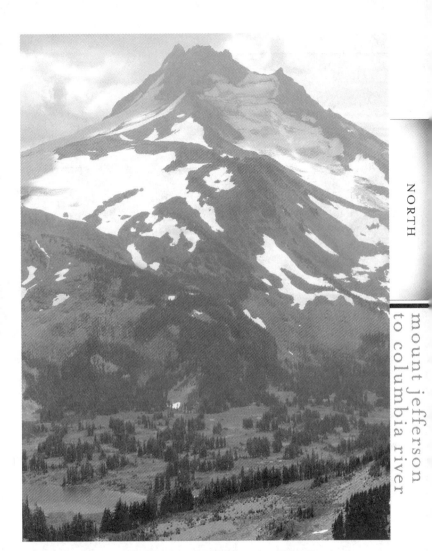

Mount Jefferson from the PCT's crossing of Park Ridge, where Hikes 18 and 19 intersect

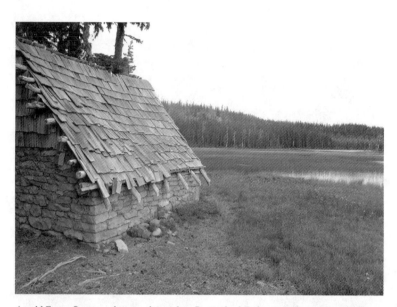

An old Forest Service cabin stands watch at Breitenbush Lake, near the trailhead.

an easy overnight with the kids, this would make a lovely spot to pitch your tent. There's another lake 0.3 mile farther up the PCT with an inferior tent site on its south side.

The last half mile of this climb is in the great wide open: rocks, snow, sky, and big views. If there's a lot of snow and you can't find a trail, look for bootprints. If there aren't any prints to guide you, aim for a notch on the ridge between two bumps; that's where the trail goes.

And what an arrival! This hike saves its best for last. As you crest the ridge and look just a few miles south toward Mount Jefferson and the meadows, trees, and lakes of Jefferson Park curled up at its feet, you'll either go silent or say something like "holy mackerel" and then stand there gawking like a fool.

Jefferson, at 10,497 feet, is Oregon's second-highest peak and the toughest to climb. One of the popular routes is right up the Jefferson Park Glacier, which from Park Butte is just right of center. Farther right is the Russell Glacier, and the one draping the left side of the peak is the Whitewater Glacier. There's another glacier, the Waldo, around the other side.

Ever-popular Jefferson Park seems to sit right at your feet, but it's a little more than a 2-mile hike during which you lose 1,200 feet of altitude. If you're determined to spend the night there (and you should—just not on a summer weekend, unless you like crowds), think about coming at it from the other direction. See the Jefferson Park hike, an easy hike of about 9 miles round-trip; from this trailhead, it's closer to 12 miles with a lot more climbing.

The PCT winds through the alpine wonder on its way from Breitenbush Lake to Park Ridge.

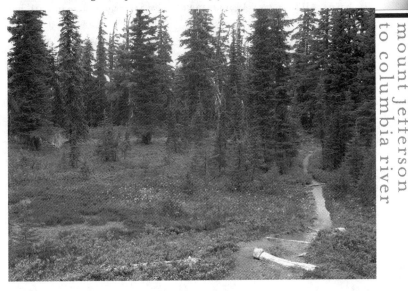

Technically, the summit of this ridge is about 200 yards west of you, a peak simply labeled "7018" on maps. The spot labeled "Park Butte" on the maps is at the end of the ridge, reached by a social trail that might make you nervous. But the view of the lakes from there is even better than here. If you're a peak bagger, knock yourself out. I'm one of the folks who'd be sitting under a tree, eating cheese and crackers, enjoying the view just like it is.

DIRECTIONS From Estacada, take OR 224 southeast for 25 miles to the ranger station at Ripplebrook. Turn south onto FS 46, and follow it for 30 miles to FS 4220, which is just before a set of power lines. Turn left onto FS 4220, Skyline Road. Or from Detroit, go 16.7 miles on FS 46 to this same intersection.

Stay right in a quarter mile, and follow the road 6.7 miles to the trailhead. This road is rough and rocky, and a lot of folks consider it a hassle. All I can say is I got my 1992 Nissan Sentra out there in 2011, but it did take 45 minutes, an average of about 8 mph.

PERMIT A Northwest Forest Pass is required for parking.

GPS Trailhead Coordinates	19 Breitenbush Lake to Park Butte
UTM Zone (WGS84)	10T
Easting	596101
Northing	495753
Latitude	N44° 45.882'
Longitude	W121° 47.135'

SCENERY: ✿ ✿ ✿	DISTANCE: *4.6 miles*
TRAIL CONDITION: ✿ ✿ ✿	HIKING TIME: *2½ hours*
CHILDREN: ✿ ✿ ✿ ✿	MAP: *Green Trails Breitenbush*
DIFFICULTY: ✿ ✿	OUTSTANDING FEATURES: *A series of moun-*
SOLITUDE: ✿ ✿ ✿	*tain lakes with occasional views of big peaks*

This casual stroll through the lovely Olallie Scenic Area visits, or comes close to, about a dozen lakes. While it might not be dramatic or challenging enough by itself to merit the long drive, the area around Olallie Lake, at this trailhead, is the perfect place to spend a weekend hiking, camping, fishing, or just lazing around. You can also start or end here and string three or four of this book's hikes together.

🚶🚶 Most thru-hikers might not even remember this section of the Pacific Crest Trail. On my thru-hike of Oregon in 2005, I ripped through here so fast I wouldn't have noticed a family of bears on the trail; that's because I had been on the trail for four days since Santiam Pass, and Olallie Lake Resort has ice cream and showers. It also has several campgrounds, cabins and boats for rent, a store, great trout fishing, and miles upon miles of trails. What I'm saying is go spend a weekend at Olallie Lake, and while you're there, check out this easy, lake-filled hike on the PCT to Upper Lake.

From the trailhead, with your store-bought coffee in hand, follow the path up a short hill to the PCT junction on a ridge above Head Lake, which has a dock for swimmers to dive from. Take a left to head north on the Crest Trail, and enjoy some nice, gradual climbing through a thin forest, with views of sprawling Olallie Lake to your left.

After a half mile, on a little bump of a hill, look behind you for a nice view of Olallie Butte, looming some 3,300 feet above the lake. A couple minutes later, arrive at a small campsite near Scharf Lake, and a minute past that, catch a view south to Mount Jefferson and a

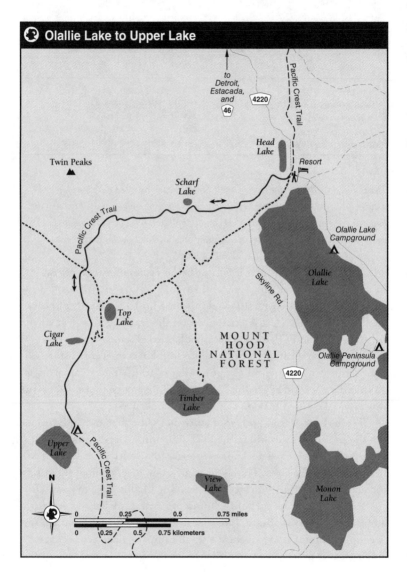

Olallie Lake to Upper Lake

to
Detroit,
Estacada,
and
46

4220

Pacific Crest Trail

Head
Lake

Resort

Twin Peaks

Scharf
Lake

Pacific Crest Trail

Olallie Lake
Campground

Olallie
Lake

Skyline Rd.

Top
Lake

MOUNT
HOOD
NATIONAL
FOREST

Cigar
Lake

Olallie Peninsula
Campground

4220

Timber
Lake

Upper
Lake

Pacific Crest Trail

N

View
Lake

Monon
Lake

| 0 | 0.25 | 0.5 | 0.75 miles |

| 0 | 0.25 | 0.5 | 0.75 kilometers |

big burned area on the far side of Olallie Lake; this 2001 burn closed a big section of the PCT between here and Mount Jefferson.

Climb for another half mile or so (but only 200 feet), and at 1.1 miles cross to the right side of a small ridge and then into a thicker forest. You pass through a saddle on the south side of a rocky peak; it's the southern half of a pair with the clever name Twin Peaks. If you're into bushwhacking, there's a small lake between them, about a quarter mile northwest of the PCT.

When the PCT drops off the saddle, you will join Trail 719, a 3-mile detour north that takes in five more lakes. Downhill, it goes to Top Lake in a quarter mile, and from there trails loops back to the resort and also visits Timber Lake. Did I mention there are a lot of lakes around here?

Staying straight ahead for Upper Lake, in a little less than a half mile you hit the southern end of the Top Lake Trail; stay to the right and uphill, and in a moment arrive at the long, thin Cigar Lake (another creative name). Beyond this lake, after a very brief climb, stroll across a meadow for 0.4 mile to Upper Lake—passing on the east side of two peaks called, yes, Double Peaks. Why can't they be named Bert and Ernie or something else?

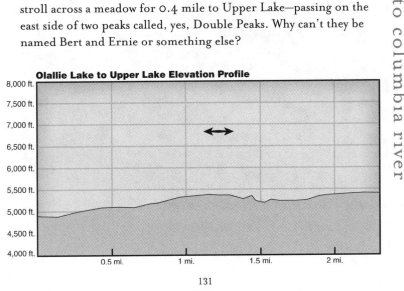

Olallie Lake to Upper Lake Elevation Profile

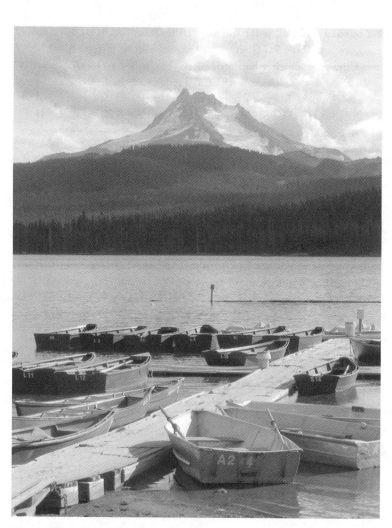

Mount Jefferson from the resort at Olallie Lake

Just as you arrive at Upper Lake, there's a nice, big campsite on the right, and halfway down the lakeshore, a trail goes left (east) a couple hundred feet to a meadow with more (but bumpy) camping. The best site, if you're looking for one, is at the far end of the lake, where a trail turns right (west) and heads around the shore. A few hundred yards up, a trail goes up and to the left (south) to a private site on a small knoll, away from the trail.

Note to the long-distance crowd: This hike lies immediately north of the Breitenbush Lake to Park Butte hike, which in turn connects to the Jefferson Park hike, which isn't terribly far from the Pamelia Lake to Shale Lake hike (Hikes 17–19). You could connect all four, starting at Olallie Lake and winding up at the Pamelia Lake Trailhead, for a total of a little less than 30 miles—a traverse of the Mount Jefferson Wilderness that would make a wonderful three- or four-day excursion.

Scharf Lake on the PCT near Olallie Lake

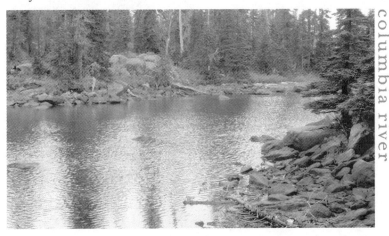

DIRECTIONS From Detroit, take FS 46 east for 25 miles to the intersection with FS 4690, where there's usually a large "Olallie" sign with an arrow painted on the road. If you're starting in the Portland area, this intersection is 45 miles from Estacada via OR 224 and FS 46, which you pick up at Ripplebrook.

Either way, turn east onto narrow but paved FS 4690. The pavement ends after 6.3 miles, and 2 miles past that, turn right onto FS 4220, which leads 5 miles to the resort entrance. To reach the PCT trailhead, stay right at the Y-junction, and look for the parking lot 100 feet ahead on the right.

PERMIT None

GPS Trailhead Coordinates	20 Olallie Lake to Upper Lake
UTM Zone (WGS84)	10T
Easting	595615
Northing	4963018
Latitude	N44° 48.850'
Longitude	W121° 47.445'

21 Little Crater Lake to Timothy Lake

SCENERY: 🐾 🐾	HIKING TIME: *2½ hours*
TRAIL CONDITION: 🐾 🐾 🐾	MAP: *Green Trails* High Rock
CHILDREN: 🐾 🐾 🐾 🐾	OUTSTANDING FEATURES: *An amazing*
DIFFICULTY: 🐾	*geological oddity, old-growth forest, a pleasant*
SOLITUDE: 🐾 🐾 🐾	*stream, and campsites on the shore of a large lake*
DISTANCE: *4.4 miles*	

Hardly a wilderness area, Timothy Lake nonetheless does have some quiet stretches and backcountry camping. This hike visits some of those and includes a trip to fascinating Little Crater Lake. If you like having a forest to yourself, a nearby section of the Pacific Crest Trail is your kind of trail.

🚶 You start out in a big, beautiful meadow that seems as though it should be filled with deer and elk, though I've never seen either one there. As for Little Crater Lake, don't think you're heading for something that even remotely resembles the famous Crater Lake. The latter is in a caldera and your destination is technically an artesian spring, which means that neither of Oregon's "crater" lakes is in a crater.

None of that matters, of course. Little Crater Lake is a jewel in a perfect setting, hidden away in a pocket of trees just 500 feet into this hike. It was formed when the earth cracked along a fault and water came up through a gravel layer to wash away soil on the surface. It's 45 feet deep, about the same distance across, and a constant 34°F.

Past the lake, follow a boardwalk over a stile and eventually through a cattle gate and into the forest. (The ground here will leave no doubt as to which side of the gate the cows live on.) It's just 0.3 mile from the trailhead to the PCT, which you join in a grove of big Douglas firs and rhododendrons. You could turn right here and

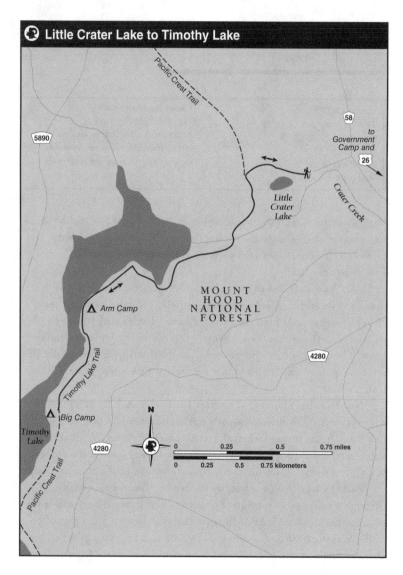

Little Crater Lake to Timothy Lake

Pacific Crest Trail

5890

58

to
Government
Camp and

26

Little
Crater
Lake

Crater Creek

MOUNT
HOOD
NATIONAL
FOREST

△ Arm Camp

4280

Timothy Lake Trail

△ Big Camp

Timothy
Lake

4280

Pacific Crest Trail

N

0   0.25   0.5   0.75 miles

0   0.25   0.5   0.75 kilometers

enjoy a 3-mile walk in the woods, which you're sure to have all to yourself. Chances are that only a PCT thru-hiker or autumn mushroom hunter would be here, but according to one guidebook, the trees here include Douglas fir; western and mountain hemlocks; western red and Alaska cedars; silver, noble, grand, and subalpine firs; and western and white lodgepole pines. It's 3 miles to FS 58, and you could make a loop by walking back down the road 3.3 miles to the trailhead. If you're thinking more long-term, it's 8 miles north on the PCT from where you've hit the PCT to US 26 near Frog Lake; that's also the start of the Twin Lakes Loop (Hike 22, page 140).

Heading south on the PCT, in 0.3 mile you come to the Timothy Lake Trail, where you turn left and, in a couple minutes, cross lovely, swift-flowing Crater Creek on a big, wide bridge. From here, the combination PCT and Timothy Lake Trail heads through a virtual tunnel of newer trees, and 0.2 mile past Crater Creek you get your first glimpse of the Timothy Lake shoreline—or, in autumn, a stump-filled marsh where the lake was in summer.

Soon the forest starts to open up a bit, the trees get older, and you are along a northeast arm of the lake. There's a campsite at 1.3

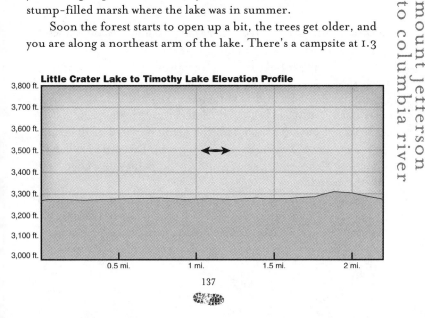

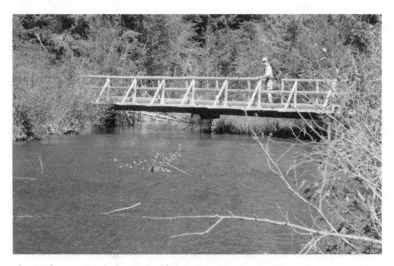

The PCT crosses Crater Creek near Timothy Lake.

miles (0.7 mile past the creek) that's away from the lakeshore; better ones lie ahead. At 1.7 miles, in fact, there's a big campsite on the shore of a little bay, and a trail leads south along the shoreline to other sites.

But the best lake access and camping are a half mile ahead, over a very small rise. When you top the hill and can see the main body of the lake through the trees, look for a faint trail leading down and to the right, toward a sprawling camping area. This place has good swimming, plenty of tent spaces, and a rocky point with a good view onto the main lake.

If you're wondering about the name Timothy Lake, it was named not for a person but for a grass. Before Portland General Electric built a dam and created the lake, a large meadow here was used for rangeland, and people sowed timothy grass to augment the food supply.

DIRECTIONS From Government Camp, go east on US 26 for 12 miles, and turn right (south) onto FS 42, following signs for Timothy Lake. Go 4.2 miles on FS 42, and turn right (west) onto Road 58, following a sign for Little Crater Lake. Turn into the Little Crater Lake Campground after 2.4 miles, and follow the access road to the parking area at the far end of the campground.

PERMIT None

GPS Trailhead Coordinates	21 Little Crater Lake to Timothy Lake
UTM Zone (WGS84)	10T
Easting	598441
Northing	5000133
Latitude	N45° 8.870'
Longitude	W121° 44.866'

mount jefferson
to columbia river

22 Twin Lakes Loop

SCENERY: 🐾 🐾	HIKING TIME: *2–5 hours*
TRAIL CONDITION: 🐾 🐾 🐾 🐾	MAPS: *USFS* Mt. Hood Wilderness or *Green*
CHILDREN: 🐾 🐾 🐾 🐾	*Trails* Mt. Wilson *and* Mt. Hood (*the lakes are*
DIFFICULTY: 🐾	*on* Mt. Wilson)
SOLITUDE: 🐾 🐾	OUTSTANDING FEATURES: *Two mountain lakes,*
DISTANCE: *4–8.5 miles*	*old-growth forest, and a nice view of Mount Hood*

There's not much of a challenge here, for either the day hiker or the overnight crowd. The total elevation gain averages less than 200 feet per mile, making this an easy-to-reach, easy-to-do introduction to the Pacific Crest Trail in the Mount Hood area. And if you want to take the family backpacking without stressing them out, this is your hike.

🏃🏃 For the PCT crowd, the Twin Lakes are a diversion used mainly for water or camping—and, even then, they're often ignored. Long-distance hikers passing through these parts are just a few miles from both a US highway and Timberline Lodge, so there's not much here for them.

In fact, this trail was originally part of the Oregon Skyline Trail and, later, the PCT, but the PCT was moved up the hill when the lakes started getting overused.

What's here for you to enjoy today are two lovely lakes and a nice viewpoint, all within easy reach. You can simply hike in to a lakeside campsite (a mere 4 round-trip miles of hiking), and in half a day you can see all the sights this area has to offer. One other suggestion before we get started: Consider combining this with the hike from Barlow Pass to Timberline Lodge (Hike 23, page 145), and you've got a one-way hike of a little less than 10 miles.

By the way, I did this hike once in mid-August in the middle of a monarch butterfly migration. It's astonishing to find hundreds of butterflies circling you. Also, the migration is fascinating, because the

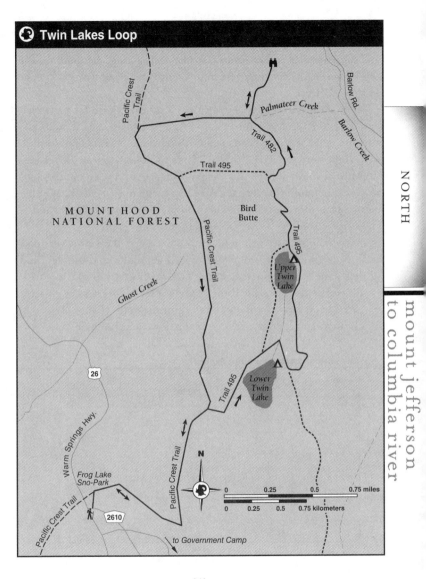

Twin Lakes Loop

Pacific Crest Trail

Palmateer Creek

Barlow Rd.

Barlow Creek

Trail 482

Trail 495

MOUNT HOOD
NATIONAL FOREST

Bird
Butte

Trail 495

Pacific Crest Trail

Ghost Creek

Upper
Twin
Lake

26

Trail 495

Lower
Twin
Lake

Warm Springs Hwy.

Frog Lake
Sno-Park

Pacific Crest Trail

N

2610

Pacific Crest Trail

to Government Camp

| 0 | 0.25 | 0.5 | 0.75 miles |

| 0 | 0.25 | 0.5 | 0.75 kilometers |

butterflies are born in California, fly to Oregon, lay eggs, and die; the ones born in Oregon then fly to Washington, lay eggs, and die; and those monarchs then fly to Canada, lay eggs, and die. Some of the ones born in Canada then return to California, often flying 100 miles in a day. Unreal.

From the parking lot at Frog Lake Sno-Park, head for the west end of the lot, and walk into the woods near a hiker sign. You'll see a picnic table, a garbage can, and two outhouses. Go 100 feet and turn right onto the PCT. Take the time to notice some evidence of the annual snowfall here: the height of the sign on your right and the blue diamond marker on a nice hemlock on the trail. That's all related to winter sports; this trail is wildly popular with the ski and snowshoe crowd for its easy access and excellent grade.

You'll appreciate that grade as you head uphill on a highway of a trail, wide enough for two people to walk shoulder-to-shoulder, and of such a mellow steepness (gaining 500 feet in 1.5 miles) that you hardly notice it—especially if the abundant huckleberries are ripe.

When you reach Trail 495, the beginning of the Twin Lakes Trail, turn right onto it, and soon drop down a hill and see Lower

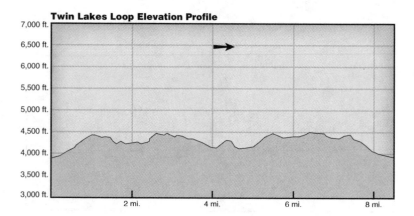

Twin Lake through the trees on your right. A social trail or two plunges down the hillside to the shore, but don't use them; they contribute to erosion, and the main trail goes to the same place. After 2 miles (and a brief trip past the lake and up a drainage), you arrive at a junction with Frog Lake Buttes Trail at the northeast shore of the lake. There's enough camping for a village here and practically nothing alive on the ground, but there's also a trail that goes all the way around the lake, leading to other campsites along the way.

To head for Upper Twin and the rest of the hike, stay on Trail 495 and you'll round a bend, climb briefly, and in 0.7 mile come to a rocky area with a view, on the left, back down to Lower Twin, pleasantly set in its steep, forested bowl. Another quarter mile brings you to Upper Twin Lake and its own round-the-lake trail. Staying on 495, go along the east side of the lake, passing a big campsite from which a small trail goes into the woods on the right—to a toilet, believe it or not. Not an outhouse, mind you, just a toilet—bizarre and quite uncomfortable looking. Upper Twin, by the way, gets less use, but that might be because it's smaller, much more shallow, and not well suited to swimming.

A half mile north of "Camp Toilet," you come to a trail on the right marked "Palmateer View." Great name, huh? Sounds like a pirate or something, but alas, it's the name of a sheepherder from pioneer days. This trail is a shortcut to Trail 482, which you reach in a few minutes; turn left there, and you'll drop down to the headwaters of Palmateer Creek (probably dry), then climb briefly to a large meadow called Palmateer Camp. From there, a moderately steep trail on the right leads a third of a mile to the viewpoint.

This view gives you a unique perspective on Mount Hood, from the southeast, and the local stretch of the PCT. It climbs this side of the ridge on your left, drops off its end to Barlow Pass, and then climbs to Timberline Lodge, the gray roof of which is visible from your viewpoint. That hike and the next section north are described here as Barlow Pass to Timberline Lodge (Hike 23, page 145) and Timberline Lodge to Paradise Park (Hike 24, page 150).

You're also looking straight across (to the north) at Barlow Butte, with meadows on the side facing you. The drainage between you and the butte is that of Barlow Creek, traced by the historic Barlow Road, which was an overland portion of the Oregon Trail used by people who didn't want to risk their lives on the Columbia River. You can still drive this road all the way to The Dalles if your car has some clearance; it's accessed just off OR 35, at the trailhead to the Barlow Pass hike.

Descending from the viewpoint, turn right onto Trail 482 at Palmateer Camp, and in 0.7 mile you are back at the PCT. You're 1.2 miles south of Barlow Pass now, but to return to your car, turn left. You'll pass the upper end of Twin Lakes Trail 495 in 0.3 mile, climb slightly for a little less than a mile, and then cruise the last 2 miles on the PCT, headed for the car. Pick some more huckleberries while you're at it. Nice and easy, huh?

DIRECTIONS From Government Camp, drive 7 miles east on US 26 to the Frog Lake Sno-Park. The trailhead is in the left-hand corner as you enter, and the sites left of it will be in the shade all day. There's car camping at Frog Lake, a half mile to the right from the parking lot.

PERMIT A Northwest Forest Pass is required.

GPS Trailhead Coordinates	22 Twin Lakes Loop
UTM Zone (WGS84)	10T
Easting	602081
Northing	5009151
Latitude	N45° 13.707'
Longitude	W121° 41.978'

23 Barlow Pass to Timberline Lodge

SCENERY: ✿ ✿ ✿	HIKING TIME: *Up to 5 hours*
TRAIL CONDITION: ✿ ✿ ✿	MAP: *USFS Mount Hood Wilderness or*
CHILDREN: ✿ ✿ ✿	*Green Trails Mount Hood*
DIFFICULTY: ✿ ✿	OUTSTANDING FEATURES: *Magnificent forest,*
SOLITUDE: ✿ ✿ ✿ ✿	*solitude, a trip to the high country, and Timberline*
DISTANCE: *Up to 10 miles, or 5 miles with a*	*Lodge*
car shuttle	

It's hard to improve on a visit to Timberline Lodge, but here are two ways: Either walk east from the lodge on the Pacific Crest Trail to some seldom-visited vistas, or climb up the trail through an amazing forest from OR 35, thus sweetening your arrival. The latter takes a second car or a 10-mile out-and-back walk, but it's the recommended route.

🚶🚶 There are more spectacular hikes in the Mount Hood area and on the Oregon PCT, but few have the combination of solitude, old-growth beauty, and mountain splendor this one has. It's also perfect for a picnic or a dose of sunshine in a high-altitude meadow with Mount Hood looming over you. And if you do the one-way option with a shuttle, you end your hike at Timberline Lodge to enjoy its food, beverages, and historic setting.

From the trailhead, walk across FS 3531 and into the woods on the PCT. Stop to admire the relief map of the trail in the area. Then take the left-most fork of the trails before you, walking north on the PCT toward Mount Hood. You take a few steps on historic Barlow Road, an overland alternative to the Columbia River back in the Oregon Trail days. After 0.1 mile along an abandoned section of the Mount Hood Highway, walk carefully across the current (and quite busy) OR 35. The trail continues in a small draw on the far side.

The first part of the trail isn't too exciting; in fact, after 0.5 mile you walk through a fairly recent clear-cut. What follows, though, is a glorious stand of noble fir, with long, straight, branchless trunks. In

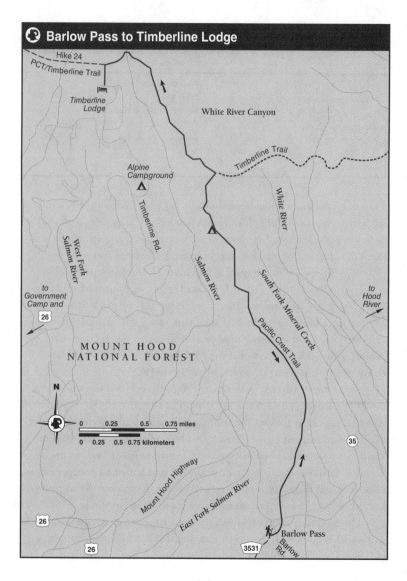

Barlow Pass to Timberline Lodge

Hike 24

PCT/Timberline Trail

Timberline Lodge

White River Canyon

Alpine Campground

Timberline Trail

Timberline Rd.

White River

West Fork Salmon River

Salmon River

South Fork Mineral Creek

to Government Camp and

26

Pacific Crest Trail

to Hood River

MOUNT HOOD
NATIONAL FOREST

N

| 0 | 0.25 | 0.5 | 0.75 miles |

| 0 | 0.25 | 0.5 | 0.75 kilometers |

35

Mount Hood Highway

26

East Fork Salmon River

26

Barlow Pass

3531

Barlow Rd.

June and July, wildflowers blanket the ground. In fall, look for huckleberries and red-and-orange vine maple. Stay quiet, especially early in the day, and you'll hear birds and possibly see deer or elk. It's just a pleasant place to be, and the trail's altitude gain (less than 400 feet per mile) is entirely manageable.

If you're wondering about those blue diamonds on the trees early in the hike, they mark winter trails for cross-country skiers and snowshoers. Their height should give you a sense of how much snow falls in these parts.

At the 2-mile mark, enter a more diverse forest, including a mix of firs and hemlocks. Cross a creek with a small campsite at 2.7 miles. Then, a little more than 3 miles out, reach an overlook of Salmon River Canyon and the headwaters of the Salmon River. The Salmon is the only river in the Lower 48 that is classified as a Wild and Scenic River from its headwaters to its mouth. The Salmon gathers its strength near the Timberline Ski Area and snakes down to the Sandy River along US 26. As you face west, note the rock patterns visible in a cliff face across the way; you're standing on layers of mudflow that burst from Mount Hood about 2,000 years ago.

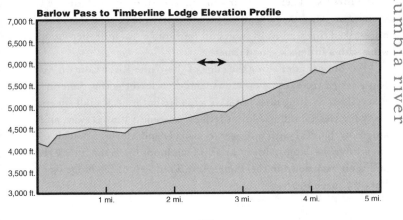

Barlow Pass to Timberline Lodge Elevation Profile

Just after this point, the forest begins to open. In July and August, enjoy meadows filled with wildflowers, especially the spectacular bear grass, which looks like a giant cotton swab. In a few minutes, reach the Timberline Trail (#600) in just such a meadow, with Mount Hood towering above you and (if it's summer) purple lupines blooming all around. For the next 20 miles or so heading north, the Timberline Trail (which goes around Mount Hood) and the PCT are one and the same.

Relax here if you'd like, and then turn around if your car is at OR 35 (for a total of 7 miles). You're at 5,300 feet elevation here (having climbed 1,100 feet since OR 35). The next 1.25 miles gain another 700 feet.

Otherwise, on you go, bearing left on the combination Timberline Trail and PCT, and in 0.3 mile find the first of several spectacular lookouts over the White River Canyon, which is 600 feet deep here. Look for buried 2,000-year-old trees in the mudflow along the far base of White River Canyon.

This section of trail is, in places, as sandy as a beach, and it tends to be windy above treeline, which can become tedious. If there's any rough weather in the vicinity, be prepared for the cold, regardless of the forecast. There's nothing to stop the wind this high on the mountain—wind that almost always blows in your face on this hike. I once hiked this section in snow and rain into a 30-mile-per-hour wind with a full pack—good times!

As you meander along the edge of the White River Canyon, you pass gnarled trees, cross meadows, and then ford the tiny Salmon River. This crossing does not have a bridge but is only ankle-deep. Look for views south to Mount Jefferson, some 45 miles away, and a sign on the PCT with mileages to Canada and Mexico. You also encounter the Mountaineer Trail, which loops up to the Silcox Hut and then back down to the Timberline Trail west of the lodge (see Hike 24, page 150).

As you approach the lodge, trails shoot off in every direction, it seems, but the PCT eventually runs into a paved road that leads down to the lodge. Or turn on your hot-chocolate radar and go for it; this is definitely a hike that finishes with style!

As I mentioned previously, it's possible to hike only the 1.5-mile upper part of this walk starting at Timberline Lodge—especially recommended if you have kids with you. This shorter option creates an easy, scenic alternative with very little elevation gain.

DIRECTIONS From Government Camp, drive 3 miles east on US 26, and then turn north on OR 35. Go 2.5 miles, and turn right onto FS 3531, following signs for Barlow Pass and the Pacific Crest Trail. The trailhead is 0.2 mile ahead on FS 3531.

PERMIT A Northwest Forest Pass is required.

	23 Barlow Pass to Timberline Lodge
GPS Trailhead Coordinates	
UTM Zone (WGS84)	10T
Easting	603107
Northing	5015159
Latitude	N45° 16.942'
Longitude	W121° 41.119'

24 Timberline Lodge
to Paradise Park

SCENERY: 🐾 🐾 🐾 🐾	HIKING TIME: 2½–7½ hours
TRAIL CONDITION: 🐾 🐾 🐾 🐾	MAP: *Geo-Graphics* Mount Hood Wilderness *or*
CHILDREN: 🐾 🐾	*Green Trails* Mount Hood/Timberline Trail
DIFFICULTY: 🐾 🐾 🐾 🐾	OUTSTANDING FEATURES: *Up-close views of*
SOLITUDE: 🐾 🐾	*Mount Hood, a dramatic canyon, wildflowers, and*
DISTANCE: *5–13 miles*	*waterfalls*

"Going through hell to get to heaven" might be a little extreme, but this is a pretty tough hike, especially since you have to cross a 600-foot-deep canyon twice. But Paradise Park is about as nice as things get in Oregon. There are shorter options here, however, and if you make it an overnight, you'll find great camping.

🚶🚶 For the Pacific Crest Trail thru-hiker, this stretch of trail is mainly about Timberline Lodge. Those words mean showers, laundry, resupply, a hot tub, and a legendary breakfast buffet. But for day hikers and overnighters, Timberline is just a starting point. Our destination is a mountainside garden of flowers, water, and stones at the foot of a mighty volcano. Either a long day hike or an easy overnight, Paradise Park will reward your efforts with pleasant walking through fantastic scenery—after you've paid the price of admission.

From the parking lot, start out on the near side of the lodge, where a big sign says it's a quarter mile up to the PCT. And by the way, don't worry if you hear blaring hip-hop and see winter clothes in the parking lot; it's just summer ski camps, bound for the Palmer Glacier. Weave through the teenagers and head on up.

Follow a paved road up to a sign that says "Canada 550, Mexico 2108." Turn toward Canada and enjoy views of Trillium Lake, Mount Jefferson, the Three Sisters, and even faraway Diamond Peak as you pass under two chairlifts and by a radio tower. There are various other

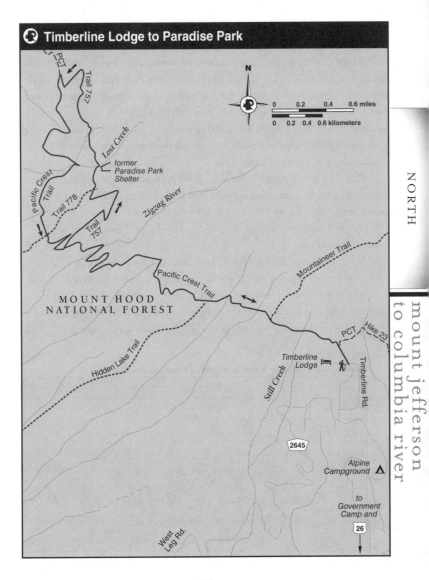

N

0   0.2   0.4   0.6 miles

0   0.2   0.4   0.6 kilometers

NORTH

PCT

Trail 757

Lost Creek

former
Paradise Park
Shelter

Pacific Crest
Trail

Trail 778

Trail
757

Zigzag River

Mountaineer Trail

Pacific Crest Trail

MOUNT HOOD
NATIONAL FOREST

Hidden Lake Trail

Still Creek

PCT

Hike 23

Timberline
Lodge

Timberline Rd.

2645

Alpine
Campground △

to
Government
Camp and

26

West
Leg Rd.

mount jefferson
to columbia river

trails and service roads that might confuse you; stay on the wide, rock-lined one heading west, and you'll be fine.

After 0.8 mile, you come to the Mountaineer Trail, which heads up to historic Silcox Hut, and a half mile past that you come to a wilderness registration station. At this point, you've gone 1.3 miles and not lost any elevation, which will soon change. By 1.6 miles, when you see the Hidden Lake Trail going down to your left, you are going ever so slightly downhill—something you may not notice until you are headed home, some 11 miles later.

But who can worry about all that when you're winding through meadows and forests, past flowers and little springs? The best of these are around 2 miles out: great vertical bands of grass and color, the farthest one with a cool view of Ski Bowl and Tom, Dick, and Harry Mountain.

Your first big Mount Hood view since the lodge is at 2.4 miles, when you reach the top of Zigzag Canyon. If you have kids or have had enough, turn around now because this canyon is something you have to go in and out of twice before the day is done, and at the bottom of it there's a river crossing without a bridge. See, straight across the

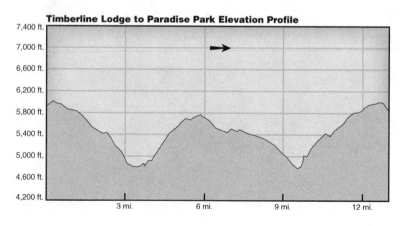

Timberline Lodge to Paradise Park Elevation Profile

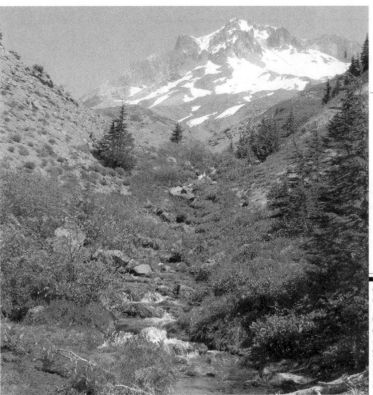

Lost Creek is just one of many scenic wonders in Paradise Park.

canyon, in a brown patch on yonder hill, a trail winding upward? That's where you're headed.

Zigzag, by the way, is a name that comes from a pioneer's description of how he traveled through here: "Turn directly to the right, go zigzag for about 100 yards, then turn short round, and go zigzag until you come under the place where you started from." You

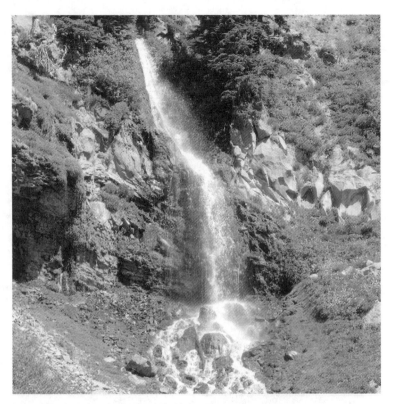

Waterfalls abound on the PCT and Timberline Trail in Paradise Park.

do something like that as you descend 600 feet on a series of switch-backs—let's call them zigzags—from the viewpoint to Zigzag River. I must offer praise to the volunteers who maintain this ever-sliding section of the trail, especially since they have to haul their tools around by hand. This section of trail also includes the only "weeping wooden wall" I can recall walking past.

When you get to the creek, you've gone 3.3 miles, and it's worth going up the creek a bit to see a waterfall farther up the canyon; I've also found the crossing up there to be better. Look around for sticks left by other hikers or cairns at good crossings—two examples of good trail etiquette.

Funny thing about this hike: You climb out of this canyon on the sunny side in both the morning and afternoon (something to think about as you start up)! After 0.7 mile, take the Paradise Park Loop Trail to the right if you want to climb up to the best attractions. If you'd like to take it a little easier, stay on the PCT for 2.1 miles to the lower end of our Paradise Park Loop, and save yourself several hundred feet of climbing.

I recommend that you head up the loop trail (#757) toward, well, paradise. Starting around 5,100 feet at the junction, hike up a side canyon to the northeast, through some intense patches of bear grass, cross a creek in a half mile, and then hike out into the clear. At a zigzag 0.1 mile later (at an elevation of 5,200 feet), look up to see the high section of trail you saw from the far side of the canyon. A left-hand zigzag is at 5,500 feet—just keeping you posted—and, 1 mile from the junction, at an elevation of 5,700 feet, you cross the Paradise Park Trail (#778). Whew!

If you're camping, there's a social trail heading up toward the peak here, and folks camp up there—just keep it under the trees, and try to limit your walking in the meadows. Call this Upper Paradise. Staying on #757, in a quarter mile you cross Lost Creek, spy an amazing campsite on a ledge above it, and a hundred yards later come to the site of the old Paradise Park Shelter, one of several built back in the 1930s for people hiking the Timberline Trail. I find it ironic that a PCT guidebook raves that this shelter once had a working fireplace—and since that was written, the shelter has burned down.

There are great campsites in this area as well, but the trail makes a right turn just before the shelter foundation and starts a long, wonderful, flat traverse through Paradise Park: heather, flowers, creeks, Mount Rainier, Mount Saint Helens, a big cliff above you called Mississippi Head, the Zigzag Glacier above that . . . not bad at all for a flat walk. After 1.2 miles of this, drop down into the forest again and intersect the PCT; this area has great views down the Sandy River Canyon, a literal cross section of Mount Hood.

To the right, the PCT starts a 3-mile, 2,200-foot drop to its crossing of the Sandy, which can be quite the adventure; I can attest that doing that section in snow and rain with a sprained ankle and a full pack is not fun. Just beyond that is Ramona Falls, which I mention only because an interesting feature of the PCT is that it gives you a new perspective on where things are in relation to each other. That is, most Oregon hikers know about Timberline Lodge and Ramona Falls, but only a PCT hiker would think about them as less than a day's walk from one another.

Turn left here, and start back toward the lodge. After an easy half mile, you come to Rushing Water Creek and its wonderful canyon, where you pass just under its waterfall; below you is an amazing slot canyon and a view down into the Sandy River Canyon. Another half mile, starting slightly downhill now, brings you back to Lost Creek. Look for a trail that leads uphill just after the crossing; it leads first to a little double waterfall and then to a magical, hidden cove with yet another waterfall. They're everywhere! It's not hard to find campsites in this area either.

Another 0.7 mile brings you to the lower end of the Paradise Park Trail, where a horse corral will encourage you to keep moving. You really head downhill now, and in 0.4 mile come back to the junction where your loop started, the Paradise Park Loop Trail, #757. Follow the PCT back down into the canyon, and, well, hate to tell you, but from here—with 9.5 miles under your belt—you've 3.5 miles to go, gaining 1,200 feet, and you've seen it all before.

But, hey, it was worth it, right? Besides, you've got Timberline Lodge to enjoy now. The hot chocolate and coffee are sublime, the food's not bad (or cheap), there's an interesting film about the lodge's construction, and its main lobby is about as nice a place to recover from a hike as you could ask for. And you deserve it.

DIRECTIONS From Government Camp, go east on US 26 for 1 mile to Timberline Rd., which leads 6 miles up to the parking lot. From the lot, walk toward the old lodge until you see the trail sign on the near side.

PERMIT A Northwest Forest Pass is required.

GPS Trailhead Coordinates	24 Timberline Lodge to Paradise Park
UTM Zone (WGS84)	10T
Easting	601041
Northing	5020512
Latitude	N45° 19.850'
Longitude	W121° 42.633'

SCENERY: ✿ ✿ ✿ ✿	HIKING TIME: *8 hours*
TRAIL CONDITION: ✿ ✿	MAP: *Geo-Graphics* Mount Hood Wilderness *or*
CHILDREN: ✿ ✿ ✿	*Green Trails* Government Camp
DIFFICULTY: ✿ ✿ ✿	OUTSTANDING FEATURES: *A historic cabin,*
SOLITUDE: ✿ ✿	*lovely waterfall, high-elevation forest, and dramatic*
DISTANCE: *13.7 miles*	*river canyon*

One part of this hike, the trip to Ramona Falls, is well known to hikers in this area. But most of the crowds headed there never make their way over to the Sandy River for the treats there.

👫 This hike starts on a trail that looks like a highway; that's because thousands of people make the trek to Ramona Falls every year. If you're looking for a quick outing or you have kids with you, consider that loop for a 7-mile excursion that won't leave you too winded.

Early in the hike, you see the results of a massive flood that occurred in November 2007. The deep cut you see here didn't exist before that day, and the trail has been moved in a few places to replace sections that are now probably down in the Columbia River. In fact, at one point about a mile up, you can see the trail reappearing on the far edge of a big bend in the gorge that wasn't there in 2006; that gives you some perspective, huh?

Just past this, 1.2 miles up, you have to cross the Sandy River, and the bridge there is only in place from mid-May to mid-October. There are often fallen trees to help you cross without the bridge, and you can wade it when it is low, but it's worth a call to the Forest Service to get the latest information.

Starting out from the trailhead, in 0.2 mile cross the Sandy River Trail, a connector from Riley Horse Camp. Keep going on Trail 797 to Ramona Falls, and admire a very large, cracked boulder

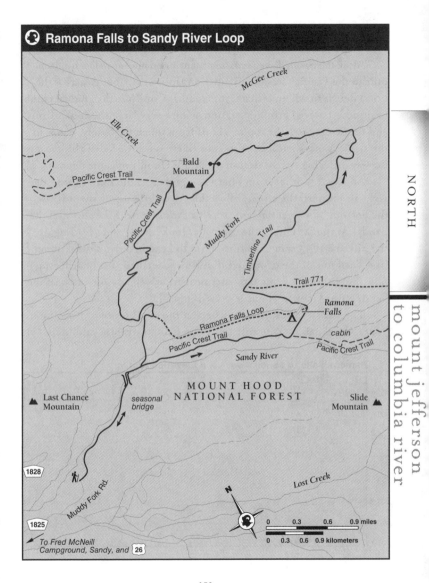

McGee Creek

Elk Creek

Pacific Crest Trail

Pacific Crest Trail

Bald Mountain

Muddy Fork

Timberline Trail

Trail 771

Ramona Falls

Ramona Falls Loop

Pacific Crest Trail

cabin

Pacific Crest Trail

Sandy River

Last Chance Mountain

seasonal bridge

MOUNT HOOD NATIONAL FOREST

Slide Mountain

1828

Muddy Fork Rd.

1825

To Fred McNeill Campground, Sandy, and 26

Lost Creek

N

| 0 | 0.3 | 0.6 | 0.9 miles |
| 0 | 0.3 | 0.6 | 0.9 kilometers |

near the junction. A short walk later, you see a nice view of Mount Hood upstream. It gets better.

After the Sandy River crossing mentioned above, walk a quarter mile to the Pacific Crest Trail junction (following ribbons across the 2007 debris flow), and turn right (south). Continue the gradual climb over moss-covered ground and under some very large rhododendrons, and 1 mile up reach the top of a bluff from which the Sandy, below to the right, is more audible. Also keep an eye out for eroded cliffs across the way, offering a cross section of Mount Hood's volcanic deposits.

An easy 1.5 miles from where you joined it, the PCT dips to the right and toward the river; follow this for a little scenic turnoff. At the bottom of a brief descent, reach a campsite near the shore of the Sandy. At the far end of the campsite, look for log steps leading up the hill to a 1935 ranger station, built to keep hikers on the Timberline Trail out of the protected Bull Run watershed. It's boarded up now, but there are some tent sites nearby, as well as a nice view of the Sandy River Canyon about 100 yards uphill.

The PCT crosses the Sandy here at the confluence of Rushing Water Creek, about 0.3 mile upstream from the cabin, and then

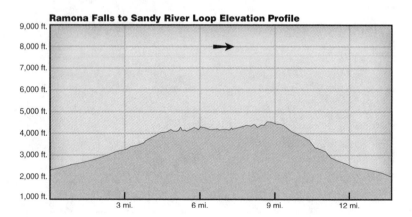

Ramona Falls to Sandy River Loop Elevation Profile

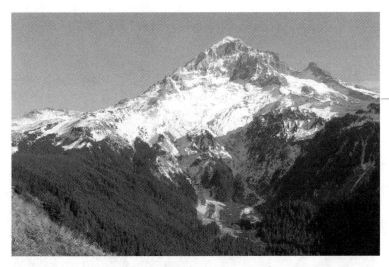

The harder return loop from Ramona Falls on the Timberline Trail lets you take in Mount Hood and the Sandy Glacier from the Bald Mountain viewpoint.

starts a long climb toward Timberline Lodge. It's worth walking out to the crossing to stand on the 2007 debris and get some amazing views up the canyon toward Hood and some big-time waterfalls. Follow more pink ribbons out here if you get confused, but be warned that they change every year because of flooding. If the campsites near the cabin are occupied, there are several nice camps along Rushing Water Creek.

Heading back now, follow the PCT back up the hill to the Ramona Falls Loop, turn right, and in 0.2 mile come to a horse gate protecting the entrance to the falls area. From here, you can drop down to the left to find campsites; camping is prohibited at the falls. Pass through the gate and enjoy yourself at the wonderful falls, which have always reminded me of one of those pyramids of champagne glasses. It's just amazing what such a small creek turns into when it falls off a cliff.

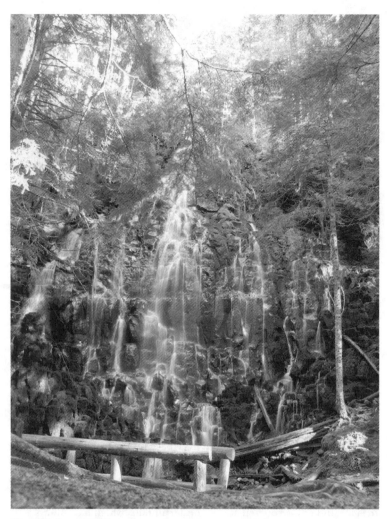

Wondrous Ramona Falls

There's a nice story, by the way, behind the naming of Ramona Falls. In 1933 a Forest Service employee came across the falls while scouting the area for a trail; at the time, he was courting his future wife and named the falls after a popular romantic song of the time named "Ramona."

Continue over the bridge and at the far end reach a junction—and a decision. You can take a simpler, shorter route back to the car or take on a big, challenging loop on the Timberline Trail, which goes around Mount Hood for 42 miles. This section used to also be the PCT, but it was rerouted because it is prone to slides and couldn't be maintained for horses. It's still a beautiful, if adventuresome, section of trail though; just call the Forest Service to check on trail conditions. I describe the two options separately below.

Going around on the Timberline Trail (9.5 miles to the car):
After climbing for 0.7 mile, reach the west end of the ridge, and find Trail 771 heading east and up Yocum Ridge. If you're curious, this trail leads 4.7 miles to a dramatic alpine landscape at an elevation of 6,200 feet at the base of the Sandy Glacier. You have to put in about 2 miles to get out of the forest. The name *Yocum,* by the way, honors an early 20th-century Mount Hood climbing guide.

From that junction, the trail becomes darn near flat, winding in and out of gullies and across small creeks. This north-facing section has snow as late as July and as early as October. After an easy 2.5 miles of this ambling, you come to the first branch of the Muddy Fork, where a small clearing on the trail includes some nice camp-sites. If you're doing this hike as an overnight, these sites are your best bet for camping.

This is also where the trail gets more entertaining, in an adventurous way. Your progress will slow as you have to pick your way through thick alder and over rocks. The trail is marked in places by rock cairns or ribbons, and the stream crossings aren't treacherous;

keep trending level and enjoy the views of Hood and the Sandy Glacier looming over you. As you look up at the mountain, the forested ridge on your left is topped by McNeil Point, a popular destination on the Timberline Trail.

At the far end of this slide area, cross the main stem of the Muddy Fork (where your feet might get a little wet), and reenter the woods in an area where damage from slides is quite apparent. Now you have an easy, viewless traverse of 2 miles to the spectacular, flower-covered lookout on the side of Bald Mountain.

A little less than a half mile past the viewpoint, you come to a major intersection of trails. The first one, on the left, is what you want: the PCT. From here, the PCT continues north to Lolo Pass, and the Timberline Trail goes back to the east and climbs toward the flowery heavens of McNeil Point, Cairn Basin, and Elk Cove.

Go south (left) on the PCT, and things get a smidge tedious, as you drop 1,500 feet in 2.3 miles of switchbacks, with nothing to see until you arrive back at the Muddy Fork. Another bridge here was destroyed, and until it's fixed you follow a diversion up and down through a swampy, cedar-filled area to the new bridge, which at least offers a parting shot of Mount Hood.

After the crossing, follow the PCT a half mile back to the junction where your loop started; cross the Sandy here and head back 1.4 miles to the trailhead.

The simpler, shorter loop (3.5 miles to the car): To complete the much simpler loop back to the parking lot from Ramona Falls, follow the trail straight ahead and down lovely Ramona Creek, perhaps singing a romantic tune as you go. It's a gently downhill 1.6 miles, featuring several log-bridge crossings of the creek, with views of fantastic rock walls on the right. See if you can spot a little section of "underground" creek as well.

When you hit the PCT, turn left and follow it for a half mile back to where your loop started. Backtrack across and then down the Sandy to your car, which is 1.4 miles down from where you hit the PCT.

A note for the long-distance crowd: This is the northernmost of four hikes in this book that trace the PCT's path past Mount Hood. You could make a fine, long hike by combining them all. Start with the Twin Lakes Loop (Hike 22, page 140), trek north onto the Barlow Pass hike to Timberline Lodge (Hike 23, page 145), keep going onto the Paradise Park hike (Hike 24, page 150), and then follow the long, pounding descent to the Sandy River.

Make that (often sketchy) crossing, and reach the site of the historic ranger cabin mentioned here. Then follow this loop around to the junction near Bald Mountain, and keep going on the PCT to the paved road at Lolo Pass. From the Twin Lakes Trailhead on US 26 to Lolo Pass, it's 26 miles one-way on the PCT. It's tough to think of a finer two- to four-day trip.

DIRECTIONS From Sandy, go east on US 26 for 17 miles to Zigzag, then turn left (north) onto Lolo Pass Rd., which is 0.6 mile past milepost 41. Go 4.2 miles and turn right onto FS 1825, which is 0.1 mile past a Mount Hood National Forest sign for "campgrounds and trailheads." Stay right at 0.7 mile, cross a bridge, and continue another 1.7 miles to turn left onto Spur Road 100, which leads 0.5 mile to the trailhead.

PERMIT A Northwest Forest Pass is required.

GPS Trailhead Coordinates	25 Ramona Falls to Sandy River Loop
UTM Zone (WGS84)	10T
Easting	591448
Northing	5026602
Latitude	N45° 23.218'
Longitude	W121° 49.910'

26 Lost Lake to Buck Peak

SCENERY: ✿ ✿ ✿	DISTANCE: *16 miles*
TRAIL CONDITION: ✿ ✿ ✿	HIKING TIME: *8 hours*
CHILDREN: ✿ ✿ ✿ ✿	MAP: *Green Trails* Mount Hood
DIFFICULTY: ✿ ✿ ✿	OUTSTANDING FEATURES: *A large lake, an old-*
SOLITUDE: ✿ ✿	*growth forest, solitude, and a mountain panorama*

Although the Pacific Crest Trail doesn't visit Lost Lake, the lake and the easy trail around it are well worth a visit. And the nearby stretch of the Crest Trail offers easy walking and remote camping in a beautiful forest, with a nice view at the end.

Like the hike from Olallie Lake to Upper Lake (Hike 20, page 129), this one is as much about the trailhead area as the PCT itself. Lost Lake, with its stocked trout and famous postcard view of Mount Hood, has camping, cabins, and boat rentals as well as an easy, 3.3-mile trail around its shore. Consider doing this hike as part of a weekend at the lake or as a fairly easy overnight backpack. You can also skip all that and park at the Huckleberry Mountain Trail, using only your Northwest Forest Pass, since that is outside the Lost Lake concessionaire's purview. Either way, this is a glimpse into what many PCT hikers experience on a trek across Oregon: easy walking through beautiful forest with almost nobody around.

Start in front of the store at the Lost Lake Resort, and look for the Lost Lake Trail heading to your right along the shore. Pass a series of picnic sites, and in a quarter mile you come to a viewing platform with a view of Hood across the way. If this particular view looks familiar, it's because you've probably seen it on a hundred calendars.

Continuing around the lake among big trees and countless huckleberries, look for a gigantic hollowed-out cedar a little less than a mile along; note that it's still alive at the top. Pass a boathouse a

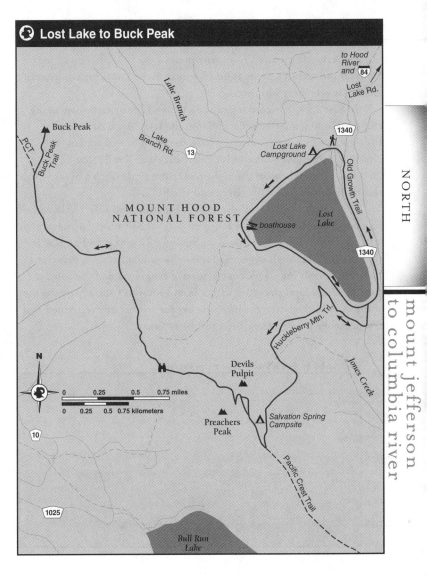

to Hood
River
and 84

Lost
Lake Rd.

Lake Branch

1340

Buck Peak

PCT

Buck Peak Trail

Lake Branch Rd. 13

Lost Lake
Campground

NORTH

MOUNT HOOD
NATIONAL FOREST

boathouse

Lost
Lake

Old Growth Trail

1340

Huckleberry Mtn. Trl.

Jones Creek

N

Devils
Pulpit

0   0.25   0.5   0.75 miles
0   0.25   0.5   0.75 kilometers

Preachers
Peak

Salvation Spring
Campsite

10

Pacific Crest Trail

1025

Bull Run
Lake

mount jefferson
to columbia river

moment later with a tiny dock on the lake; at 1.6 miles a rockslide offers a fine swimming hole. At the 2-mile mark, the unsigned Huckleberry Mountain Trail, your path to the PCT, heads up to the right. But the trail's name is odd because there's nothing in the area called Huckleberry Mountain.

In just a few moments, you see a series of poor campsites along this trail, and a quarter mile up from the lake, the trail almost touches a road before switching back to the right and starting to climb among numerous rhododendrons. After a mile that picks up 700 feet (a rockslide on the right marks the top), catch a break with a mostly flat mile to the junction with the PCT.

Turn right (north) on the PCT, and after a minute's walk come to a large campsite (which is buggy in July) at Salvation Spring, which a handwritten sign calls "Salvatoin Spring." Now the trail climbs gently for a mile through towering forest to a saddle between Preachers Peak and Devils Pulpit. A Forest Service ranger named the former for his dad, a local preacher with a bum foot who rode a horse to the summit, and the latter got its name because somebody remarked that if a preacher is here, the devil can't be far away.

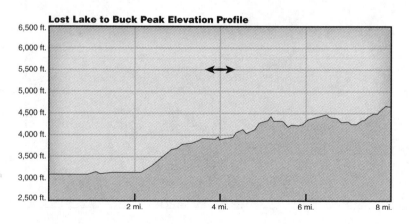

Lost Lake to Buck Peak Elevation Profile

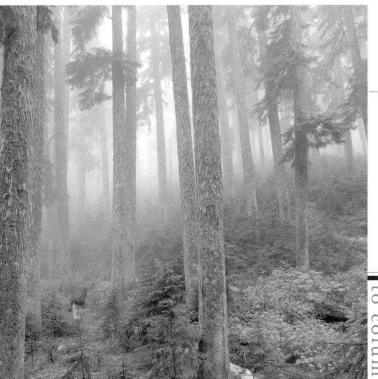

The PCT wanders through a wonderland forest above Lost Lake.

Passing between those peaks, the PCT offers views of Lost Lake and Mount Adams to the east as it loses elevation for a half mile to a rock pile on the left. Here, you can scramble up for a rare view west into Bull Run watershed, the uncut, off-limits drainage that supplies Portland with its water. From this rocky point, you can just make out Bull Run Lake off to the left.

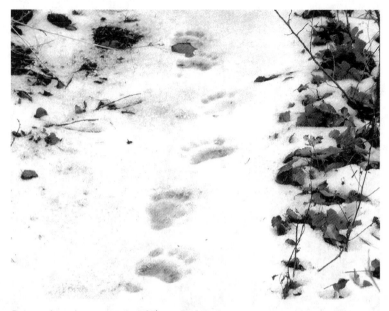

Bear tracks in the snow on the PCT near Buck Peak

At a total of 6.8 miles since the trailhead (about 2.5 miles since you got on the PCT), you round a ridge where the view north takes in a large bowl with two peaks at the far end; the one on the right is your destination, Buck Peak. Work your way around the bowl, and 1 mile north from the viewpoint, an unsigned, brushy trail heads up to the right; this is your half-mile-long summit trail.

The view from 4,751-foot Buck Peak takes in Mounts Hood, Adams, Jefferson, and Defiance (the forested one with the radio towers), as well as Lost Lake and the upper parts of the Hood River Valley. Along the summit to the left are the rusty remnants of an old lookout tower in a small meadow that makes a fine picnic site.

On your way back via Lost Lake, turn right on the round-the-lake trail and enjoy the Old Growth Trail, a boardwalk with interpretive signs about ancient forests. You can also enjoy the view from Lost Lake Butte, a 2-mile stroll that climbs 1,200 feet to a nice view of Mount Hood. Then go back to the store, and perhaps enjoy some ice cream.

DIRECTIONS From Exit 62 (west of Hood River) on Interstate 84, turn right onto Country Club Rd., following signs for several wineries. At the end of this road, 3 miles later, turn left onto Barrett Dr. Follow Barrett for 1.2 miles, and turn right onto Tucker Rd., the second stop sign you come to on Barrett Dr.

Go 2 miles up Tucker, and turn right onto Dee Hwy., where a sign says "Parkdale." After 6.5 miles on Dee Hwy., turn right again, following signs for Lost Lake. Cross a bridge, take a left onto Lost Lake Rd., and follow it for 14 miles to the resort entrance.

PERMIT The resort charges a $7 parking fee and doesn't accept a Northwest Forest Pass.

GPS Trailhead Coordinates	26 Lost Lake to Buck Peak
UTM Zone (WGS84)	10T
Easting	592317
Northing	5038742
Latitude	N45° 29.780'
Longitude	W121° 49.129'

27 Chinidere Mountain

SCENERY: ⛺ ⛺ ⛺ ⛺	DISTANCE: *4 miles*
TRAIL CONDITION: ⛺ ⛺ ⛺ ⛺	HIKING TIME: *2½ hours*
CHILDREN: ⛺ ⛺ ⛺	MAP: *Green Trails* Bonneville Dam
DIFFICULTY: ⛺ ⛺	OUTSTANDING FEATURES: *A lovely lake and*
SOLITUDE: ⛺ ⛺	*magnificent panoramic viewpoint*

If you start in Portland, you might spend more time in the car than on the trail for this one. But the view from the top of Chinidere Mountain is more than worth it, and Wahtum Lake is a fine destination as well. Still, consider making this hike a part of a longer trip to Lost Lake or the Hood River Valley or camping at the lakeside near the trailhead.

🚶🚶 If you're measuring hikes with a view-for-effort scale, Chinidere Mountain would rank an 11 out of 10—once you get there. It's almost a 2-hour drive from Portland, but it's all paved, and you'll be rewarded with a fairly easy hike, a beautiful mountain lake with camping and fishing, and a view that stretches hundreds of miles.

If you're wondering, it's pronounced "SHIH-na-dere," and it's named for the last reigning chief of the local Wasco tribe. And *Wahtum* is a Sahaptin word meaning "pond or body of water." So you're looking through the trees here at "Lake Lake."

From the trailhead, proceed through the campground (not down the road near the outhouse), and follow a trail called the Wahtum Express—so-called because it includes 250 steps. (You can skip this by following a parallel horse trail to the right, if you wish.) At the bottom of the Express, turn left and walk 100 feet down to a big tree with two Pacific Crest Trail signs on it. You are right by the lake near a picnic area and in the middle of several nice lakeshore campsites. Turn right here onto the PCT and head north.

The trail meanders along at first, near the lake, weaving through a lovely forest of hemlocks with bunchberry, thimbleberry, vanilla

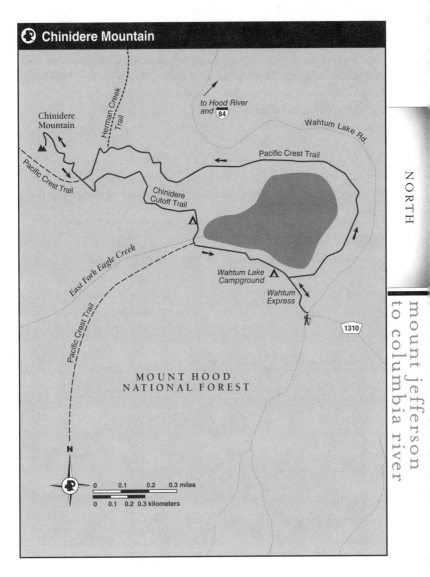

leaf, columbine, huckleberries, and salmonberry. Look along the near shore for a small island with a few trees on it. Around a half mile up there's also some impressive construction to drain water away from the trail. Tiny springs and mossy, flower-covered babbling brooks entertain and charm in a woodsy manner.

After about 1 flat mile, come into more open forest with bear grass that blooms in July, and begin climbing gradually on a classic stretch of the Oregon PCT: wide tread, soft ground, pine needles, and thick forest. At 1.75 miles, cross a creek that dries up by mid-summer, and at 1.9 miles (now having climbed 400 feet) reach the Herman Creek Trail, which leads all the way down to the outskirts of Cascade Locks.

A tenth of a mile later, look for the Chinidere Cutoff Trail (#406M), your return route, plunging down to the left. For now, go another 100 feet, and leave the PCT on the Chinidere Mountain Trail. Now you put in the climbing you've been warming up for, picking up 400 feet in a third of a mile, eventually rounding out onto the rocky summit. You might want to watch for a side trail from one of the first switchbacks, heading out into the open; it leads to

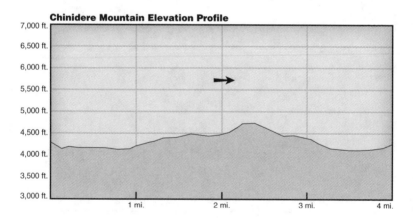

174

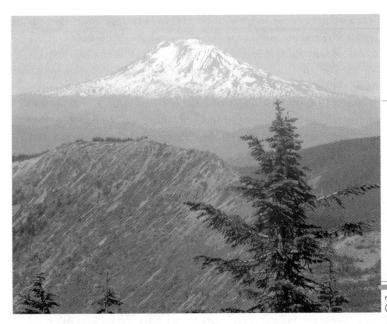
Tomlike Mountain and Mount Adams from the top of Chinidere Mountain

a rocky scramble up the west side of the mountain, which has some interesting rock benches made by industrious hikers.

After you catch your breath, soak in the view. Start by looking at Mount Hood, looming to the south. To the right of that is Mount Jefferson, and just to the left of "Jeff" is Olallie Butte. The north-bound PCT comes up the right (west) side of Jefferson, around the same side of the butte (where Olallie Lake lies), then past the right side of Hood, mostly in the trees. Just below and to the right of the summit is the Sandy Glacier, the source of the river that's such an exciting thing for hikers to cross (see the Ramona Falls description, Hike 25, page 158).

To the east, beyond Wahtum Lake, look for the upper part of Hood River Valley and to the left of that, Dalles Mountain and the desert of Central Oregon. The big peak with all the radio towers is Mount Defiance, highest spot in the Gorge, and Mount Adams is to its left. The bald ridge directly between you and Adams is Tomlike Mountain (named for Chief Chinidere's son), and left of that is the Herman Creek drainage. Off in the distance are Mounts Rainier and Saint Helens, and right in line with the latter is the broad, flat Benson Plateau. Right below you, to the west, is Eagle Creek Canyon (the East Fork drains Wahtum Lake straight away from your feet), and in the distance beyond that is Tanner Butte. On a really clear day on Chinidere, I was able to see Saddle Mountain, which is about 10 miles this side of the coast!

On its approach to Wahtum Lake, the PCT rounds an open ridge between you and Hood called Indian Mountain, and from Chinidere it heads north across the Benson Plateau and down, heinously, into Cascade Locks. But most thru-hikers take the Eagle Creek Trail—it's well graded and sports about a dozen waterfalls—then walk a few miles along the road into Cascade Locks. (All of this is described in the Eagle Creek to Benson Plateau Loop, Hike 28, page 178). After crossing the Bridge of the Gods, the trail passes the west side of Table Mountain (which looks like a big gash from Chinidere), then traces around the north side before making a swing east toward Adams, the Goat Rocks, and Rainier. So from Mount Jefferson to Mount Rainier, you're effectively looking at about 280 miles of PCT—slightly more than ten percent of it!

And by the way, the rusty cables on top of Chinidere are from an old Forest Service fire lookout, and the pits are tent sites, not vision-quest sites. Sorry it's not more romantic.

Now head back down to the PCT, turn left, and take the Chinidere Cutoff Trail, which will seem more like the Chinidere "Dropoff" Trail as it drops steeply to the lake. You cross a creek or two along the way, depending on the season, and even see a pipe along the trail that used to carry water down to some campsites on the lake's north shore. When you find these campsites, stay on the main trail, and follow it to where it crosses the East Fork of Eagle Creek on an impressive (and fun-to-cross) logjam.

Cross the creek, and in 200 yards hit the top of the Eagle Creek National Recreation Trail, which was built before 1920, connecting Wahtum Lake with the Columbia River Highway, 14 miles below. Turn left onto this trail, and follow it for about 200 hundred yards back to the PCT, which leads a quarter mile past campsites, swimming holes, and even the occasional beach. Arrive back at the bottom of the Wahtum Express—whose 250 steps will seem much less appealing to you now, no doubt.

DIRECTIONS From Interstate 84 just west of Hood River, take Exit 62, and then take an immediate right onto Country Club Rd., following signs for a bunch of wineries. At the end of Country Club Rd., 3 miles later, turn left at a stop sign onto Barrett Dr. After 1.3 miles, turn right onto Tucker Rd. (the second stop sign you come to on Country Club Rd.), which turns into Dee Hwy.

Go 8.5 miles to Dee (be sure to make a right 2 miles into this stretch, following signs for Dee and Parkdale), and turn right onto Lost Lake Rd. After 4.8 miles, turn right at a sign for Wahtum Lake onto FS 13. After 4.4 more miles, turn right again, this time onto FS 1310. Stay on the pavement for 6 miles, and then look for parking on the right. If you leave the pavement, you've gone too far.

PERMIT Parking is free for the day and $10 per night.

GPS Trailhead Coordinates	27 Chinidere Mountain
UTM Zone (WGS84)	10T
Easting	594165
Northing	5047815
Latitude	N45° 34.650'
Longitude	W121° 47.583'

28 Eagle Creek to Benson Plateau Loop

SCENERY: ♿ ♿ ♿	HIKING TIME: *2–3 days*
TRAIL CONDITION: ♿ ♿ ♿	MAP: *Green Trails* Bonneville Dam *or*
CHILDREN: ♿ ♿	*USFS* Columbia River Gorge
DIFFICULTY: ♿ ♿ ♿	OUTSTANDING FEATURES: *An amazing canyon*
SOLITUDE: ♿ ♿	*filled with waterfalls, old-growth forest, a high moun-*
DISTANCE: *29.2 miles*	*tain lake, and (farther down the trail) some solitude*

When traveling between Wahtum Lake and Cascade Locks, Pacific Crest Trail thru-hikers almost always choose the Eagle Creek Trail rather than the PCT—for reasons that will be obvious when you hike it. But why not do both? Make it a long one-nighter or casual two-nighter; it's a good early or late season getaway.

🚶🚶 Let's say you're a long-distance backpacker on the northernmost section of PCT in Oregon. You're either at Wahtum Lake, headed into the town of Cascade Locks to grab a burger, replenish your supplies, and maybe get a ride into Portland, or you're just starting your trip and heading south from Cascade Locks. Either way, you have two options: the PCT, which is steep and almost viewless, though virtually empty of humanity, and the Eagle Creek Trail, which is as crowded as anything you'll ever hike, but which includes a dozen or so waterfalls, some spectacular bridges and cliff-side trail sections, and great campsites along a splashing creek. It is, in short, one of the great trails in America.

Which would you take? Well, on this loop you'll do both; your only choice is which to do first. I prefer going up the more gradual Eagle Creek Trail and camping one night along it, then spending one night at Wahtum Lake, and leaving the dull PCT (about 16 mostly downhill miles) for the high-speed trek home.

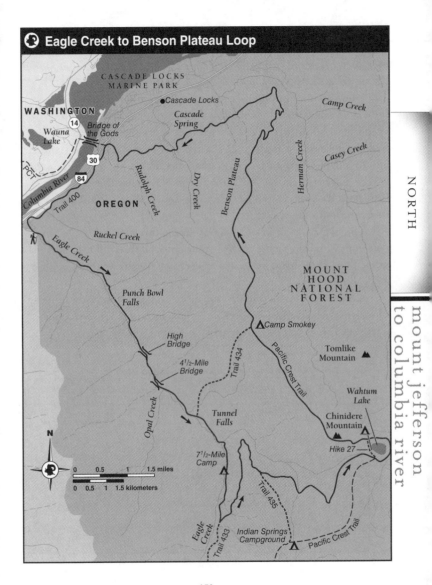

Eagle Creek to Benson Plateau Loop

CASCADE LOCKS
MARINE PARK

WASHINGTON

Cascade Locks

Cascade Spring

Camp Creek

14

Bridge of the Gods

Wauna Lake

30

84

PCT

Columbia River

Trail 400

Rudolph Creek

Dry Creek

Benson Plateau

Herman Creek

Casey Creek

OREGON

Ruckel Creek

Eagle Creek

Punch Bowl Falls

High Bridge

4½-Mile Bridge

MOUNT HOOD NATIONAL FOREST

Camp Smokey

Trail 434

Pacific Crest Trail

Tomlike Mountain

Opal Creek

Tunnel Falls

Wahtum Lake

Chinidere Mountain

Hike 27

N

0   0.5   1   1.5 miles

0   0.5   1   1.5 kilometers

7½-Mile Camp

Eagle Creek

Trail 433

Trail 435

Indian Springs Campground

Pacific Crest Trail

mount jefferson to columbia river

To do this, park at Eagle Creek, but be sure not to leave anything valuable in your car—there have been a lot of break-ins here. I don't even lock my doors at this lot, but I have an old car that no one would bother to steal.

If you're here in October or November, take a moment to look for Eagle Creek's small run of fall chinook salmon—fish that spend their adult lives in the ocean come more than 70 miles up the Columbia River, swim through the fish ladder at Bonneville Dam, and then come here to spawn. A small dam blocks their further progress up Eagle Creek, but in October and November they spawn in little round pools cleared by volunteers to simulate conditions in a wild mountain stream.

The Eagle Creek Trail is an impressive thing in itself. The work that went into it was a heroic feat: they chipped the trail into cliff faces, built High Bridge over the gorge, and hacked a tunnel behind a falls 6 miles up.

A little less than a mile up, you come to the first of several places where you walk a ledge with a cable to hang on to. If it's a summer weekend, things can get interesting here while you're trying to

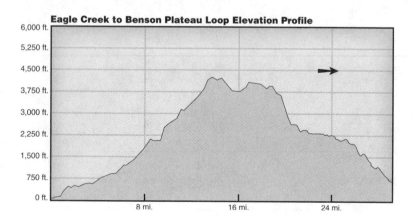

Eagle Creek to Benson Plateau Loop Elevation Profile

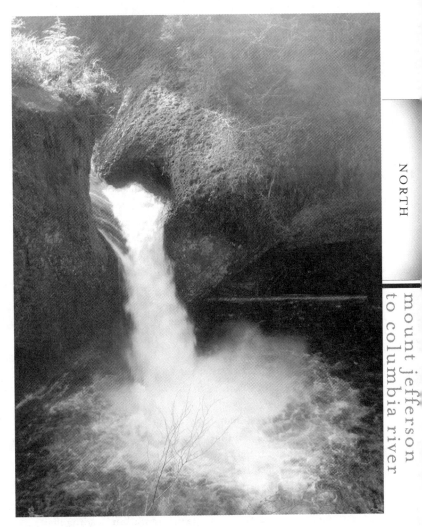

Punchbowl Falls along Eagle Creek

negotiate for cable space with dozens of other hikers. At 1.5 miles, a short side trail leads to a viewpoint of Metlako Falls (named for a native goddess of salmon), the first of many such sights of your day. Just past the viewpoint is a bench for resting. At 1.8 miles and another bench, a side trail leads down to Punch Bowl Falls, a must-see diversion and the end of the line for a lot of day hikers. Go 0.2 mile down this trail to a large clearing that's often filled with people swimming and sunbathing. At the upstream end of the clearing is a lovely (and often photographed) view of Punch Bowl Falls.

Continuing up, in 0.3 mile you get a bird's-eye view of Punch Bowl Falls; then the gorge narrows considerably. Loowit Falls is visible on the right just before High Bridge, and 0.3 mile later you come to a great picnic spot and a rare chance for access to the creek itself, in this case at the top of Skooknichuck Falls.

At 4 miles out, you cross 4½-Mile Bridge. You may wonder, what gives? Well, the fish hatchery back at the trailhead wasn't there when the trail was built (there was no need for it because Bonneville Dam didn't exist yet), so the trailhead used to be a half mile farther north, at the edge of the Columbia River Highway.

Just past the bridge, look on the right for a double waterfall, and a half mile above that, a sign explains that the area you're now entering was burned in a 1902 fire; there are still some charred stumps around. So all the trees you'll see in this area are, though large, less than 100 years old.

After 1.5 more miles, bringing your total to 6, you enter a deep gorge where Tunnel Falls plunges 130 feet and the trail goes behind it through a 35-foot tunnel. Tunnel Falls is on East Fork Eagle Creek, which drains Wahtum Lake—where you'll be later.

To see one final, dramatic falls, go about 0.2 mile farther up the trail. This falls doesn't have an official name, but it does have an interesting crisscross feature in its upper section, leading many people to call it Crisscross or Crossover Falls.

The next mile of trail is right along the creek, leading to 7½-Mile Camp, which of course is 7 miles from the trailhead. This large camping area is an excellent place to stop for your first night if you're making the loop over two nights. With a second night at Wahtum Lake or even Benson Plateau, you have plenty of time to kick around Eagle Creek. There are also some campsites between here and Wahtum Lake, which I'll point out.

Beyond the camp, the trail leaves the creek for good and starts two long switchbacks that total 3 miles and gain only 700 feet. At the end of the second switchback, you are on the northern end of a spur ridge, with a view back down the canyon. The next 1.6 miles are a bit steeper, but they end at Indian Springs Fork of Eagle Creek, where a nice campsite awaits, a total of 11 miles since the trailhead. Gradually climb for 2 more miles past wildflowers, under magnificent trees, and across splashing creeks to the shores of Wahtum Lake at the head of East Fork Eagle Creek.

Here you have another decision to make. There are campsites right and left, and the PCT is now only 0.1 mile to your right. (If you go that way, do *not* camp in the day-use area along the shore.) It's a shorter trip if you go left and the campsites are less crowded, but it's also steeper going that way. But since going right is basically recreating the Chinidere Mountain trip (Hike 27, page 172), go ahead and turn left to knock some distance off the hike. (You can still visit Chinidere going this way.)

At the lake's outlet, turn left onto the Chinidere Cutoff Trail, and skip across the logjam at the mouth of the creek. Just beyond this crossing are several campsites, in an area where a large Boy Scouts lodge burned in the 1920s. The remnants of the stone fireplace still exist to the right of the trail.

Beyond this area, the trail gets steep—some might say darn steep or even worse. It climbs 600 feet in 0.7 mile, after which you're back on the PCT. Turn left to continue your trip, and in

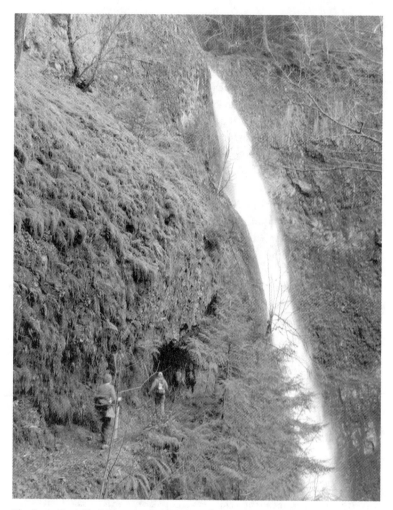

The Eagle Creek Trail enters the tunnel behind Tunnel Falls.

100 feet the Chinidere Mountain Trail takes off (and up) to your right. (For a lengthy description of this well-worth-it viewpoint, see Hike 27.)

From here, the PCT takes off north toward the Columbia River. After a mild descent along Chinidere's south side, drop through three saddles, the last of which is called Camp Smokey; as you may guess, there's a campsite here with a spring. You can also see the top end of the Eagle–Benson Trail, a legendarily steep (and very rarely maintained) cutoff back to the Eagle Creek Trail. Don't take it, except to reach a better campsite about 200 yards down it, with water 50 yards beyond that.

Leaving the camp, climb for a half mile onto Benson Plateau, named not for the famous timber man and philanthropist Simon Benson (who gave Portland its famous downtown water fountains) but for Thomas Benson, an 1864 pioneer from Missouri who lived in Cascade Locks. It is a large, completely forested plateau crisscrossed with trails. The PCT stays on its eastern edge for about 2 miles, passing several variations of Trail 405 along the way. If you want to camp on the plateau, there's a good spot with water about a half mile down Trail 405, which is the second trail you reach on the left, halfway along the edge of the plateau.

Leaving the plateau, begin a long, generally viewless descent, losing 2,700 feet over 3.4 miles to a junction with Trail 405E, which cuts 1.8 miles north to the Herman Creek Trailhead. After that junction, put in another 2.3 miles to Dry Creek, which isn't, and immediately past that cross a road you can follow 0.2 mile left to see a 50-foot waterfall.

Truly getting back into civilization now, head 0.7 mile to a power-line road, walk along it for 70 yards, and then pick up the PCT for a 1-mile descent to Trail 400, the Gorge Trail. If you're winding up in Cascade Locks, stay on the PCT for a final 0.1 mile, and you end up in the parking lot for the Bridge of the Gods—

mount jefferson to columbia river

which, by the way, is how PCT thru-hikers get over the Columbia, believe it or not. If you're coming out at Eagle Creek, turn left on Trail 400, which more or less parallels Interstate 84 for 2.5 miles back to the Eagle Creek Trailhead.

DIRECTIONS From Portland on Interstate 84, drive 34 miles east of Interstate 205, and take Exit 41 for Eagle Creek. Go 0.2 mile, turn right, and continue 0.6 mile to the end of the road. If it's crowded, you might have to park closer to the highway and hike that much farther.

PERMIT A Northwest Forest Pass is required at Eagle Creek.

GPS Trailhead Coordinates 28 Eagle Creek
to Benson Plateau Loop

UTM Zone (WGS84) 10T
Easting 583862
Northing 5054601
Latitude N45° 38.393'
Longitude W121° 55.435'

Appendix A: Hikes by Category

Day Out-and-Backs
(some may also be overnights)

1 California Border to Observation Peak
2 Grouse Gap to Siskiyou Peak
3 OR 99 to Pilot Rock
5 OR 62 to Pumice Flat
6 OR 62 to Crater Lake Rim
7 Crater Lake Rim
10 Rosary Lakes to Maiden Peak Shelter
14 Lava Camp Lake to Collier Glacier View
15 Little Belknap Crater
18 Jefferson Park
19 Breitenbush Lake to Park Butte
20 Olallie Lake to Upper Lake
21 Little Crater Lake to Timothy Lake
23 Barlow Pass to Timberline Lodge
26 Lost Lake to Buck Peak

Day Loops
(some may also be overnights)

4 Sky Lakes Wilderness
16 Three-Fingered Jack
22 Twin Lakes Loop
24 Timberline Lodge to Paradise Park
25 Ramona Falls to Sandy River Loop
27 Chinidere Mountain

Overnight Hikes
(some may also be done as day hikes)

4 Sky Lakes Wilderness
6 OR 62 to Crater Lake Rim
8 Mount Thielsen Loop
9 Tipsoo Peak and Maidu Lake
10 Rosary Lakes to Maiden Peak Shelter
11 Mink Lake Basin
12 Wickiup Plain to Sisters Mirror Lake
13 Obsidian Loop
14 Lava Camp Lake to Collier Glacier View
16 Three-Fingered Jack
17 Pamelia Lake to Shale Lake Loop
18 Jefferson Park
19 Breitenbush Lake to Park Butte
22 Twin Lakes Loop
24 Timberline Lodge to Paradise Park
25 Ramona Falls to Sandy River Loop
26 Lost Lake to Buck Peak
28 Eagle Creek to Benson Plateau Loop

Appendix B: Contacts

BUREAU OF LAND MANAGEMENT
www.blm.gov

Medford District
www.blm.gov/or/districts/
medford/index.htm
3040 Biddle Road
Medford, OR 97504
(541) 618-2200

COLUMBIA RIVER GORGE
NATIONAL SCENIC AREA
www.fs.usda.gov/crgnsa
902 Wasco Street, Suite 200
Hood River, OR 97031
(541) 308-1700

CRATER LAKE NATIONAL PARK
www.nps.gov/crla

Supervisor's Office
P.O. Box 7
Crater Lake, OR 97604
(541) 594-3000

DESCHUTES NATIONAL FOREST
www.fs.usda.gov/centraloregon

Supervisor's Office
1001 SW Emkay Drive
Bend, OR 97702
(541) 383-5300

**Bend–Fort Rock Ranger
District**
1230 NE Third Street,

Suite A-262
Bend, OR 97701
(541) 383-4000

Crescent Ranger District
136471 Highway 97 N
Crescent, OR 97733
(541) 433-3200

Sisters Ranger District
Pine Street and Highway 20
Sisters, OR 97759
(541) 549-7700

MOUNT HOOD NATIONAL FOREST
www.fs.fed.us/r6/mthood

Supervisor's Office
16400 Champion Way
Sandy, OR 97055
(503) 668-1700

**Clackamas River Ranger
District**
595 NW Industrial Way
Estacada, OR 97023
(503) 630-6861

Hood River Ranger District
6780 Highway 35
Parkdale, OR 97041
(541) 352-6002

Zigzag Ranger District
70220 East Highway 26
Zigzag, OR 97049
(503) 622-3191

Pacific Crest Trail Association
www.pcta.org

1331 Garden Highway
Sacramento, CA 95833
Office: (916) 285-1846
Trail conditions (toll-free):
(888) 728-7245

Rogue River–Siskiyou National Forest
www.fs.usda.gov/rogue-siskiyou

Supervisor's Office
3040 Biddle Road
Medford, OR 97504
(541) 618-2200

High Cascades Ranger District
www.fs.usda.gov/detail/
rogue-siskiyou/about-forest/
offices#highcascades
47201 Highway 62
Prospect, OR 97536
(541) 560-3400

Siskiyou Mountains Ranger District
www.fs.usda.gov/detail/
rogue-siskiyou/about-forest/
offices#highcascades
6941 Upper Applegate Road
Jacksonville, OR 97530
(541) 899-3800

Umpqua National Forest
www.fs.usda.gov/umpqua

Supervisor's Office
2900 NW Stewart Parkway
Roseburg, OR 97470
(541) 957-3200

Diamond Lake Ranger District
2020 Toketee RS Road
Idleyld Park, OR 97447
(541) 498-2531

US Forest Service: Pacific Northwest Region
www.fs.fed.us/r6
333 SW First Avenue
Portland, OR 97208
(503) 808-2468

Willamette National Forest
www.fs.usda.gov/willamette

Supervisor's Office
3106 Pierce Parkway, Suite D
Springfield, OR 97477
(541) 225-6300

Detroit Ranger District
P.O. Box 320
Mill City, OR 97360
(503) 854-3366

McKenzie River Ranger District
57600 McKenzie Highway
McKenzie Bridge, OR 97413
(541) 822-3381

contacts

Appendix C: Hike Agencies

Note: See agencies in Appendix B for specific contact information.

SOUTH: *California Border to Mount Thielsen*

1. California Border to Observation Peak: Siskiyou Mountains District (Rogue River–Siskiyou National Forest)

2. Grouse Gap to Siskiyou Peak: Siskiyou Mountains District (Rogue River–Siskiyou National Forest)

3. OR 99 to Pilot Rock: Medford District (Bureau of Land Management)

4. Sky Lakes Wilderness: High Cascades Ranger District (Rogue River–Siskiyou National Forest)

5. OR 62 to Pumice Flat: Crater Lake National Park

6. OR 62 to Crater Lake Rim: Crater Lake National Park

7. Crater Lake Rim: Crater Lake National Park

8. Mount Thielsen Loop: Diamond Lake Ranger District (Umpqua National Forest)

9. Tipsoo Peak and Maidu Lake: Diamond Lake Ranger District (Umpqua National Forest)

CENTRAL: *Willamette Pass to Santiam Pass*

10. Rosary Lakes to Maiden Peak Shelter: Crescent Ranger District (Deschutes National Forest)

11. Mink Lake Basin: Sisters Ranger District

12. Wickiup Plain to Sisters Mirror Lake: Sisters Ranger District (Deschutes National Forest)

13. Obsidian Loop: McKenzie River District (Deschutes National Forest)

14 Lava Camp Lake to Collier Glacier View: Sisters Ranger District
    (Deschutes National Forest)

15 Little Belknap Crater: Sisters Ranger District
    (Deschutes National Forest)

16 Three-Fingered Jack: Sisters Ranger District
    (Deschutes National Forest)

NORTH: *Mount Jefferson to Columbia River*

17 Pamelia Lake to Shale Lake Loop: Detroit Ranger District
    (Willamette National Forest)

18 Jefferson Park: Detroit Ranger District
    (Willamette National Forest)

19 Breitenbush Lake to Park Butte: Clackamas River Ranger District
    (Mount Hood National Forest)

20 Olallie Lake to Upper Lake: Clackamas River Ranger District
    (Mount Hood National Forest)

21 Little Crater Lake to Timothy Lake: Clackamas River Ranger
    District (Mount Hood National Forest)

22 Twin Lakes Loop: Hood River Ranger District (Mount Hood
    National Forest)

23 Barlow Pass to Timberline Lodge: Hood River Ranger District
    (Mount Hood National Forest)

24 Timberline Lodge to Paradise Park: Zigzag Ranger District
    (Mount Hood National Forest)

25 Ramona Falls to Sandy River Loop: Zigzag Ranger District
    (Mount Hood National Forest)

26 Lost Lake to Buck Peak: Hood River Ranger District (Mount Hood
    National Forest)

27 Chinidere Mountain: Columbia River Gorge National Scenic Area

28 Eagle Creek to Benson Plateau Loop: Columbia River Gorge
    National Scenic Area

hike agencies

Index

Adventure Medical first-aid kits, 9
animals
   approaching, 17
   and plant hazards, 11–14
Atwater Carey first-aid kits, 9

backcountry advice, 15–17
Bald Mountain, 164, 165
Barlow Creek, 144
Barlow Pass, 140
Barlow Pass to Timberline Lodge,
      145–149
bathrooms, 16–17
Bays Lake, 119
bears, 12–13
Benson, Simon, 185
Benson, Thomas, 185
Benson Plateau Loop from Eagle
      Creek, 178–186
best-maintained trails,
      top five, xv
Black Butte, 106
Black Crater, 100
Bonneville Dam, 180, 182
boots for hiking, 7–8
Breitenbush Hot Springs, 120–121
Breitenbush Lake, 118, 121, 133
Breitenbush Lake to Park Butte,
      122–128
Bridge of the Gods, Cascade Locks,
      20, 185–186
Broken Top, 76
Buck Peak from Lost Lake,
      166–171
Bull Run Lake, 169

calderas, 54
California border to Observation
      Peak, 20–24
Camelot Lake, 83
Canyon Creek, 104, 107
Cascade Locks, 20, 174, 176, 178,
      185, 185–186
Cascade-Siskiyou National
      Monument, 32
Cathedral Rocks, 114
central Pacific Crest Trail hikes,
      70–107
children
   hiking with, 9
   top five hikes for, xv
children (hike profile), 4
Chinidere, Chief, 176
Chinidere Mountain, 172–177
Cigar Lake, 131
Cliff Lake, 78, 79
clothing for hiking, 7–8
Coffin Mountain, 96
Collier Glacier, 85, 97, 101
Collier Glacier View from Lava Camp
      Lake, 92–97
Crater Creek, 137
Crater Lake, 39
Crater Lake Lodge, 46
Crater Lake National Park, 42
Crater Lake Rim, 52–57
Crater Lake Rim from OR 62, 47–51
Crater Peak, 45

Dalles Mountain, 176
deer ticks, 11–12

Detroit Lake, 96
Devils Lake, 84, 85
Devils Peak, 39, 55
Devils Pulpit, 168
Diamond Lake, 57, 60, 64
Diamond Peak, 150
difficulty (hike profile), 4
difficult hikes (most), top five hikes,
    xvi
Dilldock Pass, 91
distance (hike profile), 4
dog ticks, 11–12
dogs, top five hikes for, xvi
Donomore Meadows, 20
Double Peaks, 131
drinking water, 6–7, 10
Dumbbell Lake, 78
Dutchman's Peak, 22
Dutton Creek, 49

Eagle Creek National Recreation
    Trail, 177
Eagle Creek to Benson Plateau Loop,
    178–186
easy hikes, top five, xv
elevation profiles, 2
Elk Lake, 91
Elk Lake Resort, 80
emergencies
    animal, plant hazards, 11–14
    first-aid kits, 8–9
    general safety, 9–11
    hypothermia, 11
equipment, essential, 8
etiquette, trail, 17
Eugene Chapter (Oregon Nordic
    Club), 74

fires, 15–16
first-aid kits, 8–9
flat hikes, top five, xvi

food, 10, 16
footwear for hiking, 7–8
Frog Lake, 137, 142

garbage, 15, 17
Garmin GPS units, 1–2
Giardia (waterborne parasite), 6–7
Goat Rocks, 176
Gorge, the, 176
GPS trailhead coordinates, 2–3
Grizzly Peak, 112
Grouse Gap to Siskiyou Peak,
    25–29
guidebook, using this, 1–4

Head Lake, 129
Heavenly Twin Lakes, 36
High Bridge, 182
hike profiles, 3–5
hikes. *See also specific hike*
    from CA border to Mount
        Thielsen, 19–69
    Mount Jefferson to Columbia
        River, 108–186
    star ratings, 4–5
    top five by category, xv–xvi
    Willamette Pass to Santiam Pass,
        70–107
hiking
    backcountry advice, 15–17
    with children, 9
    clothing for, 7–8
    safety, 9–11
    ten essentials for, 8
    tips for enjoying PCT in Oregon,
        14–15
    trail etiquette, 17
    weather, 5–6
hiking time (hike profile), 4
Hillman Peak, 49, 56–57

Hinch, Stephen, 3
Hood River, 170
House Rock, The, 84
Howlock Mountain, 66
Hunts Cove, 114
Hunts Lake, 114
hypothermia, 11

Indian Mountain, 176
Jack Creek, 107
Jack Lake, 102
Jefferson, Thomas, 23
Jefferson Park, 116–121
Jefferson Park Glacier, 127

key, and overview map, 1
Klamath Lake, 38
Kokostick Butte, 81
Koosah Mountain, 81, 83

Lake of the Woods, 114
Lancelot Lake, 83
latitude/longitude coordinates, 2
Lava Camp Lake, 86
Lava Camp Lake to Collier Glacier
    View, 92–97
Le Conte Crater, 84, 85
Lee Peak, 39
Lewis and Clark's Corps of Discovery,
    121
Linton Meadows, 86, 88
Little Belknap Crater, 92, 98–101
Little Brother, 90
Little Crater Lake to Timothy Lake,
    135–139
Lolo Pass, 165
longitude/latitude coordinates, 2
Lost Creek, 155, 156
Lost Lake Butte, 171
Lost Lake Resort, 166
Lost Lake to Buck Peak, 166–171

Lower Rosary Lake, 72
Lower Twin Lake, 143
Luther Mountain, 38

Mac Lake, 79
Maiden Peak Saddle, 74
Maiden Peak Shelter from Rosary
    Lakes, 72–75
map (hike profile), 4
maps. *See also specific hike*
    central Pacific Crest Trail, 70
    northern Pacific Crest Trail, 108
    overview, key, 1
    southern Pacific Crest Trail, 18
    topographic, 2
    trail, 1
Marble Mountains, 23
Marguerette Lake, 38, 41
Mazama Village, 49
McKenzie Pass, 91, 98
McNeil Point, 164
Merrill Lake, 79
Mesa Creek, 85
Metlako Falls, 182
Middle Rosary Lake, 74
Middle Sister, 67, 88, 97, 100, 101
Milk Creek Canyon, 112
Miller Lake, 68
Mink Lake Basin, 76–80
Minnie Scott Spring, 96
Mississippi Head, 156
Moraine Lake, 83
mosquitoes, 14
Mount Adams, 96, 169, 170, 176
Mount Ashland, 33
Mount Bachelor, 67, 76
Mount Defiance, 170
Mount Hood, 121, 143, 145, 148,
    152, 160, 164, 165, 166, 170,
    171, 175
Mount Hood Chapter (PCTA), 122

INDEX

Mount Jefferson, 62, 92, 110, 112,
    114, 116, 121, 122, 124, 126–127,
    129, 131, 148, 150, 170, 175, 176
Mount Jefferson to Columbia River
    hikes, 108–186
Mount Mazama, 46, 54
Mount McLoughlin, 23, 35, 39, 54,
    62
Mount Rainier, 156, 176
Mount Saint Helens, 156, 176
Mount Shasta, 35, 39, 55, 62
Mount Thielsen, 27, 56, 57, 61, 66,
    67, 101
Mount Thielsen Loop, 58–63
Mount Washington, 92, 101
mountain lions, 13
Muddy Fork, 164

National Geographic's TOPO maps, 1
navigation equipment, 8
North Matthieu Lake, 91, 92
North Rosary Lake, 74
North Sister, 88, 92, 97, 100, 101
North Umpqua River, 68
northern Pacific Crest Trail hikes,
    108–186

Observation Peak from California
    border, 20–24
Obsidian Falls, 88
Obsidian Loop, 86–91
Odell Lake, 72
Olallie Butte, 175
Olallie Lake Resort, 129
Olallie Lake to Upper Lake,
    129–134
Opie Dilldock Pass, 90–91, 96–97
OR 62 to Crater Lake Rim, 47–51
OR 62 to Pumice Flat, 42–46
OR 99 to Pilot Rock, 30–35

Oregon Geographical Names, 22
Oregon Mule Skinners, 122
Oregon Nordic Club
    (Eugene Chapter), 74
Oregon Skyline Trail, 140
Outdoor Navigation with GPS (Hinch), 3
outstanding features (hike profile), 4
overview map, 1

Pacific Crest Trail
    central hikes, 70–107
    northern hikes, 108–186
    southern hikes, 19–69
    tips for enjoying, 14–15
    weather, 5–6
Pacific Crest Trail Association,
    Mount Hood Chapter, 122
Palmer Glacier, 150
Pamelia Lake, 118, 133
Pamelia Lake to Shale Lake Loop,
    110–115
Paradise Park from Timberline Lodge,
    150–157
parasites, waterborne, 6–7
Park Butte, 119, 127, 128
Park Butte from Breitenbush Lake,
    122–128
Phantom Ship, Crater Lake, 62
Pilot Rock, 27
Pilot Rock from OR 99, 30–35
plant, animal hazards, 11–14
poison ivy, oak, sumac, 13–14
Porcupine Rock, 106
Porky Lake, 80
Portland General Electric, 138
Portland's average temperature, by
    month (table), 6
Preachers Peak, 168
Pumice Flat from OR 62, 42–46
Punch Bowl Falls, 182

Ramona Falls, 156
Ramona Falls to Sandy River Loop,
    158–165
Red Cone, 68
Riley Horse Camp, 158
Rim Village, 54
Rock Mesa, 84
Rosary Lakes to Maiden Peak Shelter,
    72–75
Rushing Water Creek, 156, 160, 161
Russell Glacier, 127
Russell Lake, 119

S Lake, 79
Saddle Mountain, 176
safety
    first-aid kits, 8–9
    tips, 9–11
Salmon River, 147
Salvation Spring, 168
Sandy Glacier, 163, 175
Sandy River Canyon, 156
Sandy River Loop from Ramona Falls,
    158–165
Santiam Pass, 122, 129
Sawtooth Ridge, 66
scenery (hike profile), 4
scenic hikes, top five, xv
Scharf Lake, 129
Scout Lake, 119
Sentinel Hills, 116
Shale Lake, 110, 112, 114, 118
Shale Lake Loop from Pamelia Lake,
    110–115
shield volcanoes, 101
shoes for hiking, 7–8
Silcox Hut, 152
Sink Creek, 81
Siskiyou Mountains, 25
Siskiyou Peak from Grouse Gap,
    25–29

Sister Spring, 88
Sisters Mirror Lake from Wickiup
    Plain, 81–85
ski trips, top five hikes, xvi
Skooknichuck Falls, 182
Sky King Cole Ranch, 32
Sky Lakes Wilderness, 36–41
snakes, 12
snowshoes, top five hikes for, xvi
solitude (hike profile), 4
solitude, top five hikes for, xv
South Fork Breitenbush River, 120
South Matthieu Lake, 91, 92
South Sister, 67, 76, 79, 81, 84
southern Pacific Crest Trail hikes,
    19–69
star ratings, 4
steepness, top five hikes for, xvi
streams, crossing, 10
Stuart Falls, 45, 46

Table, The, 114
Table Mountain, 176
temperature, Portland's average by
    month (table), 6
Thielsen Creek, 57, 64
Three Sisters, 55, 57, 150
Three Sisters Wilderness, 76
Three-Fingered Jack, 101, 102–107
ticks, 11–12
Timber Lake, 131
Timberline Lodge, 140
Timberline Lodge from Barlow Pass,
    145–149
Timberline Lodge to Paradise Park,
    150–157
Timothy Lake from Little Crater Lake,
    135–139
Tipsoo Peak, 62
Tipsoo Peak and Maidu Lake, 64–68
toilets, 16–17

Tom, Dick, and Harry Mountain, 152
Tomlike Mountain, 176
topographic maps, 2
trail condition (hike profile), 4
trail etiquette, 17
trails. *See also* hikes *or specific hike*
    maps, 1
    staying on, 10
Trapper Lake, 38
trash, 15, 17
Trillium Lake, 150
Tunnel Falls, 182
Twin Lakes Loop, 140–144
Twin Peaks, 131

Union Peak, 44, 45
Upper Lake, 166
Upper Lake from Olallie Lake,
    129–134
Upper Snow Lakes, 40
Upper Twin Lake, 143
UTM (Universal Transverse Mercator)
    coordinates, 2–3

volcanoes, shield, 101

Wahtum Lake, 172, 176, 177, 178, 182,
    183

Wasco Indians, 172
Wasco Lake, 102, 104, 106
Watchman, The, 55, 56
Watchman Peak, 49
water, drinking, 6–7, 10
weather, 5–6
West Cascade Chapter, Backcountry
    Horsemen of Oregon, 122
West Nile virus, and mosquitoes, 14
White Branch Creek, 90
White River Canyon, 148
Whitewater Glacier, 127
Wickiup Plain to Sisters Mirror Lake,
    81–85
Wife, The, 84
wildflowers, top five hikes for, xvi
wildlife, top five hikes for, xvi
Willamette Pass to Santiam Pass hikes,
    70–107
Willamette Stone State Heritage Site,
    28
winter, top five hikes in, xvi
Wizard Island, Crater Lake, 55

Yapoah Crater, 92
Yocum Ridge, 163

Zigzag Canyon, 152–154
Zigzag Glacier, 156

About the Author

One day, PAUL GERALD was sitting in his cubicle at a highly respected insurance company when the phone rang. It was a good friend inviting him on a walk across Oregon on the Pacific Crest Trail. A few months later, Paul was unemployed and sleeping in the woods—just the way he likes it.

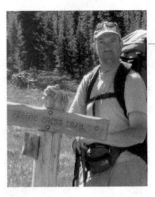

It's not like he was a "career guy" when that phone rang. He grew up in Memphis and developed addictions early on to both hiking and traveling. He got the journalism bug while at Southern Methodist University in the 1980s and went on to work in the sports departments of the *Dallas Times-Herald* and *Memphis Commercial Appeal*. He was also a staff writer for the *Memphis Flyer*, and to this day, some 15 years and three hundred columns later, he remains their travel writer. He moved to Portland in 1996 because it's a whole lot closer to mountains, old forests, clear rivers, and lonesome ocean beaches. Along the way, he has also written for Portland's *Willamette Week*, the *Oregonian*, and all sorts of newspapers, magazines, and websites around the country. And to avoid doing any settled kind of work, he has also dabbled in commercial fishing, landscaping, social work, the YMCA, tossing packages into trucks, and an amusement park.

Today, he is still a freelance writer specializing in his three passions— food, the outdoors, and travel. He is also the author of Menasha Ridge Press's *60 Hikes within 60 Miles: Portland*, the fourth edition of which came out in spring 2010. In 2008 and 2010 he wrote and published *Breakfast in Bridgetown: The Definitive Guide to Portland's Favorite Meal*. Paul is also the executive director of the Northwest Association of Book Publishers and an employee of Embark Adventures, a Portland-based international adventure travel company.

To keep up with Paul and get in touch with him, stop by and visit **www.paulgerald.com**.

Taking care of the Pacific Crest Trail is a full-time effort.

The Pacific Crest Trail Association's mission is to protect, preserve and promote the trail as a resource for hikers and equestrians and for the value that wild lands provide to all people.

Through a formal partnership with the U.S. Forest Service, our nonprofit membership organization is the primary caretaker of this 2,650-mile National Scenic Trail as it winds through the American West's most beautiful landscapes.

Each year, PCTA volunteers and paid staff members clear downed trees and repair washed out tread. We monitor threats to the trail and speak up on its behalf. We tell the trail's story in print and online. And we advocate for federal support by visiting our elected leaders in Washington, D.C.

All this effort safeguards the experiences and solitude people deserve when they venture into the wild.

Please help preserve this national treasure for future generations by joining the PCTA.

Your $35 annual membership will ensure that this trail will never end.

Photo by Josh Meier

1331 Garden Highway
Sacramento, CA 95833
(916) 285-1846
www.pcta.org • info@pcta.org

PACIFIC CREST TRAIL
ASSOCIATION